GABRIELA ROSA, MScM (RHHG), BHSc (ND)

FERTILITY
BREAKTHROUGH

Overcoming infertility and
recurrent miscarriage when other
treatments have failed

ALL AUTHOR ROYALTIES ARE
DONATED TO THE ROSA FOUNDATION
FOR FERTILITY RESEARCH.

RETHINK PRESS

BREAKTHROUGH

\ 'brāk-ˌthrü \ noun

An act or instance of moving
through or beyond an obstacle*

* Merriam-Webster dictionary definition.

For my patients, who taught me how to unconditionally love long before the birth of my own children, and who inspire me every day with their courage and strength.

PRAISE

'In her new book *Fertility Breakthrough*, Gabriela Rosa gifts men and women faced with the daunting challenge of infertility with her holistic and science-based blueprint optimising the potential for a successful pregnancy. Blending wit and wisdom, *Fertility Breakthrough* provides the reader with Gabriela's tips, tools and techniques based upon her years of experience guiding couples desperately seeking trusted guidance.'

Dr Pamela M. Peeke, MD, MPH, FACP, FACSM
New York Times bestselling author of *Body for Life for Women*,
Assistant Professor of Medicine, University of Maryland, USA

'Reproductive medicine is an ever-evolving field. Through clinical research, patient education and technological advancements couples who in the past may perhaps never otherwise had conceived or had the opportunity to experience a healthy full term pregnancy, will become parents. For many, Gabriela Rosa is the reason. I have known and worked closely with Gabriela for over twenty years and I have been privileged to witness first-hand the passion and devotion with which she approaches the care of her patients. *Fertility Breakthrough* is a compilation of over two decades of clinical experience in helping couples become parents. A must read for anyone who wishes to improve their chances of delivering a healthy baby.'

Dr James Ferry, MBChB, FRANZCOG, FRACGP
Obstetrician and Gynaecologist, Senior Lecturer at University of
Sydney Medical School and Notre Dame School of Medicine,
Head of Obstetrics Department at Mater Hospital

'*Fertility Breakthrough* is a must read for anyone who is ready to embrace an integrative approach to addressing their struggle to achieve a successful pregnancy outcome. In her book, Gabriela Rosa delivers an effective action plan that she has created and carefully refined over her many years helping thousands of couples navigate the often bewildering spectrum of fertility options. To any couple desperately seeking fertility help, *Fertility Breakthrough* is a welcome relief.'

Dr John Demartini
Internationally bestselling author of *The Values Factor*

'Gabriela Rosa's *Fertility Breakthrough* makes a meritorious contribution to future generations of healthy children, whose parents will have benefited from her comprehensive body of work. I love how Gabriela provides her patients and readers with the necessary education to understand how to take responsibility for their own health, as well as inspiring through her extensive expertise and valuable advice the understanding that emotional and physical well-being must be equally revered when the goal is to live a whole and fulfilled life.'

Pete Evans
Celebrity chef and Producer of *The Magic Pill*

'Gabriela Rosa's new book *Fertility Breakthrough* is a very welcome addition to the growing body of evidence that acknowledges the essential truth that fertility is multifactorial. She gives clear guidance on the many factors that can either enhance or impair fertility, and dispels many myths which can cause unnecessary heartbreak for so many couples experiencing difficulties. Over the many years I have known and worked with Gabriela, I have always been impressed with her dedication to her work, her thorough approach and her boundless enthusiasm. Read this excellent book and you will also be impressed, enthused and optimistic about your ability to improve your fertility and conceive a healthy baby.'

Francesca Naish

Internationally bestselling author of *Natural Fertility*, *The Natural Way to Better Babies*, *Better Pregnancy*, *Better Birth and Bonding*, and *Better Breastfeeding*

'Throughout *Fertility Breakthrough*, Gabriela Rosa lovingly guides readers through her multifaceted, holistic approach to fertility treatment. She educates and empowers couples to take control of their own health and well-being as a foundational approach to increase the potential of a successful pregnancy and healthy baby. Well done, Gabriela. May this become the first resort for all couples who want a healthy baby.'

Narelle Chenery

Co-founder and Creative Director of Miessence

'Our evolutionary bodies (that's right they are not modern) need certain ingredients – real food, sunshine, sleep, connection, clean water and movement – as the basics in order to express health. Infertility and miscarriage occur not because of one thing; there are many things. It's about looking at the body as a whole and not just testes, ovaries and uterus. Gabriela Rosa's book *Fertility Breakthrough* brings you back to what's important, to explore the root cause of a complex issue and empower individuals and couples to take complete charge of their life and health. This book will not only help with a successful pregnancy but improve the chances of a healthy child.'

Cyndi O'Meara

Nutritionist, Founder of Changing Habits, and Producer of *What's with Wheat?*

'Gabriela Rosa has invested decades to develop and continuously fine tune an approach to fertility treatment that is a much-needed paradigm shift for couples experiencing reproductive challenges. As a scientist, I am concerned with adequate methods to reach effective results, and in Gabriela's latest book, *Fertility Breakthrough*, couples will find a comprehensive, scientific, evidence-based guide to understanding how to change their results. Gabriela's book speaks to the core of why many couples may struggle for years to have a baby, but most importantly how they can take matters in their own hands to overcome all previous difficulty and reach their most desired outcome of a healthy baby. I wholeheartedly recommend Gabriela's work to couples all over the world.'

Dr Leticia Kawano-Dourado, MD, PhD
Clinical Research Scientist, University of São Paulo Medical School, Brazil

'Nothing ever goes away
until it teaches us
what we need to know.'
Pema Chödrön

CONTENTS

PART 2 – FROM CHALLENGE TO BREAKTHROUGH   77

FOREWORD

Four years. Forty-eight menstrual cycles. Forty-eight 'two-week waits'. Forty-eight silent, body-shaking, heart-wrenching sobbings in the shower, run hot to hide the swollen redness of my distraught face from my husband.

We did everything we knew how to do – standard therapy, non-conventional methods, seemingly everything – and we still weren't pregnant. *Why?* We'd had no trouble getting pregnant with our first son, and when he was two years old, we wanted to be pregnant again. We had conceived him after only three months of trying. Now, we wanted to complete our family. We researched, we prayed, we wondered. Our heads spun, trying to understand.

As a paediatric and pregnancy chiropractor, I have extensive training in and professional study and practice on the nervous system, endocrine and immune systems. My husband, a spinal rehabilitative corrective chiropractor, is also extensively trained and equally health focused in how we live our lives. Anyone who knew us would say we were the healthiest couple they could think of. So, why weren't we pregnant?

Surely we weren't alone. Through our research, we found that one in six couples struggle with infertility worldwide. One in four women and one in four men have a primary factor creating an inability to conceive. Like many of these people, we went to the internet several times to seek guidance on this journey but became overwhelmed by all the conflicting information and advice available.

One particular spring day, the Alaskan sun that was shining through my window was in direct contrast to the torrential storms I felt in my heart. I had been weeping and just sat in front of my computer, lost as to which direction to go. I could barely make out a prayer: 'Please, please. I have no idea what to do. I've done all I can. I know you have put it in my heart to have another child, and I know you have the power to help. I will accept your will, but I have to do all I can first. Please, please. Guide me.'

When I opened my eyes, the sun was still bright, and now I felt peace in my heart. I typed something on Google and Gabriela's website stood out. I opened it. At first I was sceptical, but then I read her qualifications and consumed all the information she provided freely. I realised that despite everything I knew, Gabriela already had a track record and experience along two decades in helping couples in my very situation. I was tired of the 'get pregnant fast' schemes. I knew anything I pitched to my husband would have to have some serious research and clout behind it, so I scheduled a phone call to Gabriela's team alone to do some scouting, and prayed he'd be open to listening, too.

I don't know what I was expecting, but Gabriela got me to do more work and answer more questions before I so much as spoke to her than I had been asked to do in four years of struggling through infertility. I thought, 'Finally, someone is listening!' Gabriela had an effective process to determine if we were a good match for working together. I was impressed. When she said that we wouldn't even be trying for a baby for at least four to six months, and given our specific circumstances it could even be closer to a year, I was disheartened. But when I understood the 'why' behind those recommendations, I was ready to comply. I feel like most of us have very few 'whatever it takes', 'all or nothing' moments or decisions to act upon in our lives.

Creating a healthy human being doesn't command as many accolades as, say, starting a billion-dollar empire from scratch, winning a Nobel Prize or finding a cure to a rare disease. But I would venture a guess that for those of us who have suffered the pain of infertility through years of disappointment and heartbreak, none of those earthly accomplishments would bring as much joy as the simple and quiet 'positive' on a home pregnancy test.

We decided that we would do 'whatever it took'.

We committed to ourselves and we gave it our all. Was it easy? By no means. It took dedication, patience, tears, frustration and even more patience. It took pain, anger, laughter and suffering. But the support and guidance were amazing, and with it we stayed the course. And in due time and with much work, that unique moment of looking at my positive pregnancy test became a reality once more. I had an elaborate plan as to how I was going to share the news with my husband, but I ruined it all by laughing and jumping up and down while on the phone with our local doctor, who confirmed, based on my human chorionic gonadotropin (hCG) numbers, that I was truly pregnant.

We wanted our son, Isaius, to be the first to know about the pregnancy. On the day of his sixth birthday, we took him to our twenty-week ultrasound. The sonographer turned on the machine and an image of his sister popped up. We said, 'Happy birthday, buddy! Do you know what that is?' He said, in his sweet, squeaky six-year-old voice, 'Is that a baby? *It's a baby! Mom!* You're going to have a baby? I'm a *big brother!*' We could hardly contain our joy, and gave him the job of telling the rest of our families.

A few months later, our beautiful daughter Isliana was born, six and a half years after her brother. To see the two of them is like seeing my very own fertility puzzle made whole. They were truly made for each other. The first words out of his mouth when he saw her were, 'I prayed for her. Mom, you did great work.' To this day, even though sometimes he remembers 'the good old days when it was just Mom, Dad, and me – before my baby sister destroyed my Legos', he loves that he's a big brother and our family is complete.

All the pain, tears, suffering and sorrow were replaced with elation, happiness and a quiet peace that fills my soul. 'Whatever it takes', with God's will and Gabriela's team, was enough for us. Gabriela was kind to remind us that no matter what happened, we needed to be happy right where we were. That way of considering life and its challenges, including this one, in and of itself brought me perspective. Gabriela and her team do not promise the world, but to my family and me, they over-delivered in terms of helping me find myself and my strength again along my struggles. And as I see baby after baby after baby being born to those under her care, I see in each the miracle of an answered prayer, as it was for me.

I encourage you to feast upon Gabriela's work. Use highlighters, take notes, come back again and again to soak up her wisdom and evidence-based prescriptions, which give life to the words she shares in this book. Whether you use this book simply, as one of Gabriela's recommendations suggests, to live your best life now or to improve your current chances of getting pregnant, I know the fact that you're holding this book is already a blessing. Now it's up to you. Be sure to put it to good use.

Dr Jessica J. Dachowski
Anchorage, Alaska (USA), 2019

INTRODUCTION

'Now is the time to understand more,
so that we may fear less.'

Marie Curie

Some couples get pregnant easily, others don't. Many struggle to take a healthy pregnancy to full term and deliver a healthy baby. In fact, it takes one in six couples longer than twelve months to get pregnant, leading to an infertility diagnosis.[1,2] And one in five known pregnancies end in miscarriage.[3,4]

Reproduction is still one of the areas in which most people feel disempowered when things don't go immediately to plan. Technology has left us feeling powerful. We control what and when our groceries get delivered. We control what piece of content we consume at any given time. We control our banking and finances at the touch of a button on our phone. But biology has received no updates from the App Store in millions of years. Yet, our expectations regarding our body's capabilities continue to escalate.

Technology is shaping our lives in ways we couldn't have imagined a few short years ago. It plays a part in our increased prosperity and improved education opportunities, as well as our health and longevity.[5]

On the other hand, it seems this extra 'availability' of everything we need has reduced our ability to think critically and be confident fact-finders. Our access to the curated lives of others leads us to believe fertility is a given. Google has replaced qualified health advice, as we search for quick solutions to complex issues; and Facebook has become the 'place to be' as we share more and disclose less. Could it be that as we become more connected with the rest of the world, we become less connected with what we need to thrive?

Our expectations have changed – we want it now, at the lowest possible cost, with minimum or, even better, *no* effort. We want the silver bullet, preferably in the form of the smallest number of pills possible. We chase the quick fix and drown in an ever-expanding ocean of misinformation. In my work with tens of thousands of patients, I have seen, with growing concern, the worrying trend of unfulfilled reproductive expectations, despite the scientific and medical breakthroughs. In a world where you can get practically everything on demand, optimum fertility is one stark exception.

Again, technology has changed us and our expectations of our lives, but our biology remains the same... You have just as much control over how long it takes for the egg to mature (about eight months) and the sperm to form (a minimum of four months) as you do over the fact that a full, healthy human pregnancy is, and has always been, nine months long. As much as we wish to advance the human body through science, we still can't hack or 'game' biology. We need to understand that as much as we can work with, nurture, support and care for our bodies by removing the obstacles to optimum health, and that these actions can help us create the miracle of life, we can't make our biology bend to our will. Especially if we choose not to remove the obstacles of modern life, which obstruct the path of homeostatic balance and thus block optimum fertility.

This book is your chance to begin to identify and remove the roadblocks on your journey to parenthood. Effectively implementing what you learn will allow you to unobstruct your path to baby, no matter how long you've been trying and what else hasn't worked. Ultimately, only you can take charge of transforming your results. Through the powerful combination of education and the inspired call to action you now hold in your hands, you now have the vehicle.

JOURNEY TO PARENTHOOD

END RESULT
LIBERATION

STEADFASTNESS
DETERMINATION
MOTIVATION

CHOICE

PROGRESS
INCUBATION
TREATMENT

CHOICE

CHOICE

CHOICE

RECOMMENDATIONS
EDUCATION
FACT FINDING

SUFFERING
HOPELESSNESS
DESPAIR

NO RESULT

No matter the circumstances that have led you to finding this book, whether you've been trying to conceive for countless years and/or have had multiple miscarriages, the information within these pages constitutes the powerful fundamentals I've used in combination with a complete strategy to help my patients overcome infertility and miscarriage, even when other treatments have failed. Trust me when I urge you to take notice, dig deeper and, most importantly, apply what I'll share with you for your and your prospective child's ultimate benefit.

Optimum reproductive outcomes rest upon a complex biochemical matrix. Thus, expecting to solve infertility and recurrent miscarriages with a quick Google search on the right supplements to take and the right diet to follow to improve your chances of having a baby is at best unrealistic and at worst, unfortunately (as I've seen happen to many couples over the years), the perfect way to continue going around in circles, only to run out of time altogether. This is especially true for couples who have been trying to have a baby for over two years, because the biological reality is that the longer you've been trying to conceive, without the right strategy on your side, the less likely you are to have a baby – without having to invest in costly and, in many cases for couples in this situation, questionably effective interventions.

In my experience over the last two decades, if a couple is categorically committed to doing whatever it takes to have a baby – no matter the challenges they may face – and they're willing to let go of preconceived notions of how specifically this will happen, they will find a way. But this will never happen if you don't become definitively clear about what you truly want (as well as why) and about what your relationship with your partner can withstand along this journey. You need to be explicitly aware of and fully prepared to make the sacrifices, as well as identify the price (physical, emotional and financial) that you're prepared to pay to achieve your outcome – this includes drawing your imaginary *finish line*. With the help of the exercises in this book, you'll also be encouraged to look inside and find your strength to arrive at the clarity of your convictions, for the sake of your own happiness and personal fulfilment – all while doing what it takes to co-create your baby.

Finally, during our time together, I'll teach you how to use my seven-step F.E.R.T.I.L.E. Method® and the 11 Pillars of Fertility Foundations™ for your ultimate benefit. This is the same proven methodology I've shared with over 100,000 people in more than 100 countries. As we work together here, you'll have every opportunity to understand exactly what it takes to leave nothing to chance and no stone unturned in making your parenthood dream come true. I am honoured to be your guide on this journey. Let me hold your hand from beginning to baby and beyond. Let's go.

References

1   Oakley, L., et al., Lifetime prevalence of infertility and infertility treatment in the UK: Results from a population-based survey of reproduction. *Hum Reprod*, 2008. 23(2).

2   Mascarenhas, M.N., et al., National, regional, and global trends in infertility prevalence since 1990: A systematic analysis of 277 health surveys. *PLoS Med*, 2012. 9(12).

3   Maconochie, N., et al., Risk factors for first trimester miscarriage – results from a UK-population-based case-control study. *BJOG*, 2007. 114(2).

4   Savitz, D.A., et al., Epidemiologic measures of the course and outcome of pregnancy. *Epidemiol Rev*, 2002. 24(2).

5   Botella, C., et al., The present and future of positive technologies. *Cyberpsychology, Behavior and Social Networking*, 2012. 15(2).

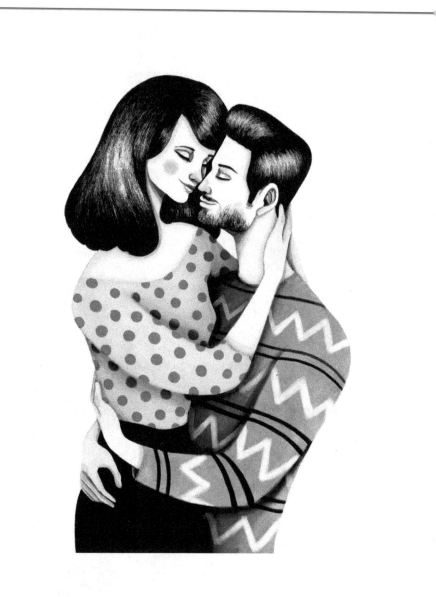

PART 1

WILL YOU EVER HAVE YOUR BABY?

'I will not be triumphed over.'

Cleopatra

M y story started when I was eighteen years old. My periods had stopped and I was worried about what was going on. I went to my doctor and explained my symptoms, and he was convinced I was pregnant.

I wasn't. I'd done multiple pregnancy tests.

Yet, he claimed, 'Every woman is pregnant until proven otherwise', and insisted on blood tests to prove himself right.

I was upset. I wasn't being heard.

My concerns, dismissed – and beneath it all, I was afraid. Petrified, actually, because I was in touch with my body and I knew something wasn't right, but I didn't know what, or what it meant. I now realise that was my first taste of, and a slight variation on, a theme my patients frustratingly endure throughout their (often prolonged) fertility journey – typically for many years.

Three days after having the requested blood tests, I called to get my results and without ceremony was told over the phone, 'You have polycystic ovary disease.'

I was panic-stricken. I have a disease? Am I going to die? What's happening?

He went on to tell me, 'Well, you'll probably never have kids. It's the number one cause of infertility in women.' And that was how my journey began.

At the time I wasn't focused on getting pregnant, but I knew that one day I wanted to have kids. It wasn't until a few years later, after I'd met my husband-to-be and began working in clinical practice, helping couples overcome infertility, that it hit me – what if I really can't have children? I didn't consciously choose to help couples overcome infertility because of my early diagnosis, but looking back now, I can see my career choices were in part how I sought to learn and help myself along the way.

Decades have passed, and to this day, I can honestly say my patients continue to be my greatest teachers. Working to learn how to best serve them, I learned a lot about how to improve my own chances of conceiving. For many years I had irregular periods, and there were many years when I had none. Yet, because of the heartache and emotional pain of my patients on their fertility journeys, the thought I might never have children was never far from my mind either.

My husband-to-be was supportive and eased my worries with his attitude. But – call it a hazard of the profession – as a fertility specialist, I liked having advance warning of what I needed to look out for in my patients' cases, and I decided being personally proactive wouldn't be a bad idea. We had only been going out for six months when I convinced him it would be a good idea to get a semen analysis. I didn't expect it to uncover any issues. After all, he was healthy and athletic (despite being ten years older), and neither of us was ready to start trying to conceive anyway. Luckily, he's also the proactive type. He agreed immediately, had the test done and, before I knew it, I was staring at the report, facing the true magnitude of the fertility problem in my/our hands.

The results of his semen analysis weren't good. The count was slightly down and the morphology (shape) of the sperm was completely abnormal at 0% (the World Health Organization guide-line expects at least 4% morphology for a man to effect a healthy pregnancy, even through in vitro fertilisation (IVF), let alone natural conception),[1] and there was also a high level of DNA fragmentation. I'd successfully treated these types of cases (many times) though, and we weren't planning on having children just yet, so after the initial shock, we got on with our lives – being very aware of our daily choices to ensure we were optimising our health and fertility.

Six years into our relationship (and two years before we wanted to start trying for a family), we decided it was time to put some concerted effort into optimising our health and fertility – despite our both pretty much living the lifestyle I recommend to my patients and implementing my own 11 Pillars of Fertility Foundations™. I still had to do some work on regulating my cycles and ovulation, and sperm quality still needed more attention. Luckily, I knew exactly what needed to be done because by then, I had already done this a few thousand times with my patients. I started taking the herbal medicines and nutrients I needed, and finally my periods became more regular. We gave our bodies the time necessary to implement everything I teach my patients to increase our chances of creating a healthy pregnancy to term and a healthy baby.

With several major 'minor factors' (see 'The Minor Things To Major In' in Part 1 for the eye-opening statistics on the effects of minor factors on your fertility) against us (my polycystic ovarian syndrome and subclinical hypothyroidism and my husband's sperm-quality issues – count, morphology and excessive DNA fragmentation), our odds of conceiving were dismal at best (according to the current statistical models applied to reproductive outcomes). However, just like my patients, I'd done the work, and after fourteen years of wondering if I'd ever be able to have a baby, I was shocked when I became pregnant on our first attempt.

Nine months later, in 2012 in Sydney, Australia, we had our first son – the highly energetic, gregarious, persistent Jake.

When I held Jake for the first time, the thought that came to my mind was 'Do your part and the Heavens will come to your aid'.

It had happened for so many of my patients before me. I was incredibly clear that this blessing had come as a result of our taking charge of our health and fertility, as well as our accepting nothing less than to leave no stone unturned and nothing to chance.

I opted for no contraception after Jake's birth. In our situation, I didn't see the point. Jake was breastfed until nineteen months, and then I knew I had to stop because my periods still hadn't returned and (unfortunately) there were no delightful 'surprises'. I wanted one more child to complete our family. Six months after I stopped breastfeeding, my periods were still nowhere to be seen, even though I was doing everything I needed to do from a lifestyle perspective.

It was the first time I truly felt and completely understood the real heartache of secondary infertility. I think as a professional, I was trained to always lead with empathy, and I never quite realised until this moment that only a woman with a negative test who wants to be pregnant 'months or years ago' truly understands this feeling – and as much as she might try to help her partner understand, its magnitude will never quite be felt in the same way. It also dawned on me at that time that empathy was helpful, but experience was my greatest teacher regarding what my patients really go through.

I'll admit, before this, the thought 'surely you'll be happy with one child' had crossed my mind many times – but the truth is that the exasperation that's so easy to feel throughout the fertility journey is difficult to put into words until one has 'been there'.

So, back I went to square one in preparing and implementing what I now refer to as the F.E.R.T.I.L.E. Method®. It took another seventeen months of preparation, six of which were intense work, to develop a predictable cycle and ovulation pattern again. I was hopeful that I'd have the same 'surprise' experience again. I'd never stopped doing my best, so surely, we'd get pregnant quickly – I hoped.

But it was a tough year and a half, filled with the same worries and great lessons. And now, I also had an extra question: 'Will my child ever have a sibling?' At some point within this time it dawned on me – I had to stop focusing on what I didn't have and what wasn't happening. I needed to do what made me happy and live my best life now, not 'at some point in the future, when I x, y, z'. The experience of not getting pregnant when I wanted taught me so much about *every* area of my life.

Over the years, I'd also seen too many people wish their lives away in this mindset of 'when I have a (or another) baby, everything will be perfect'. I was determined to enjoy my present and the gift of my life, with all the wonderful people and experiences it already contained – rather than feed that unrealistic fantasy (or, better yet, completely incorrect assumption) that everything would be perfect 'one fine day'.

I asked myself, 'What do I need most right now?' And the almost-immediate answer was 'Grounding'.

I needed something to keep my interest and attention in the present moment in a fun and creative way – and something totally different from the conversations I had all day at work. So, I decided to take up... quilting and wool appliqué.

This was the absolute highlight of my 'infertility' and I made some beautiful, wise friends to boot. My heart is filled with gratitude for the choices, experiences and flag posts along the way that helped me embrace equanimity on my fertility journey. My life has been made all the better for the understanding that no storm lasts forever and that in the middle of every storm, it's possible to keep the faith, do what it takes, and even enjoy the ride.

When my cycles finally resumed (my husband and I had taken a good dose of my/our own medicine) and my body was once again ready, we ended up conceiving on our second attempt. For the second and last time, nine months later, in 2015 in Sydney, Australia, my second son – the wise, serious and yet incredibly funny Josh completed our little family.

Since 2001, I've been holding my patients' hands from beginning to baby, to help them overcome all sorts of reasons for infertility and miscarriage. This makes me believe the same could be possible for you. And now is exactly the right time.

CHAPTER 1

There Is No Such Thing As The Perfect Time

'Everybody's at war with different things
I'm at war with my own heart sometimes.'

Tupac Shakur

Before I was thinking about having a family, I felt as if my life stretched out in front of me, full of possibilities, and that I had years to get things right. I was fortunate that I took action before it was too late, but many people are stuck in this wishful-thinking phase, assuming they have all the time in the world – that 'it will happen when it's meant to' or that it's simply 'God's will'. Personally, I believe that God (in whatever form or denomination God takes for you) helps those who help themselves.

Let's put our reproductive years into perspective. Imagine you'll live until age ninety. Now visualise your life as a series of circles. Each circle is one month of your life, and a full row of circles is three years.

LIFE IN MONTHS

(EACH ROW IS 36 MONTHS = 3 YEARS)

BIRTH

PUBERTY

PEAK
FERTILITY

PERI
MENOPAUSE

MENOPAUSE

TURNING 90

While it might seem that our lives are made up of endless months, weeks and days, they are easily countable, and finite. Take a look at a 'typical' Western woman's life choices and fertility window.

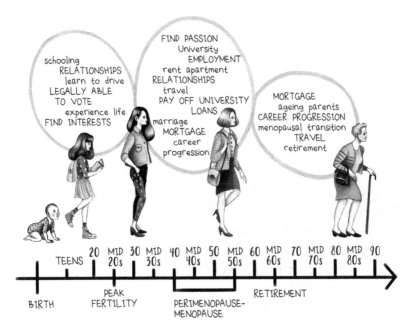

A girl's first menstrual period usually occurs between ages eleven and thirteen, although this depends on each girl, and recent research suggests that this age is decreasing in response to the Westernisation of our environments, which also means menopause is arriving earlier than usual for many women.[2,3] After puberty, female fertility increases, and then decreases. A woman's fertility peaks in her mid-twenties, after which it starts to decline slowly. Perimenopause and menopause generally occur between ages forty and fifty. Menopause is marked by the cessation of ovulation, menstruation and the end of one's natural reproductive life (although, these days, this has been extended through the use of donor egg and donor embryo technologies).

Let's see how this natural progression works with the archetypical Western woman's busy lifestyle. At age twenty-four, after attending college or university, she'll find her first job. She'll be legally allowed to drink alcohol and vote. She'll get her first car, rent her first apartment, pay off university loans, and make the first and last payments on the mortgage for her home. She'll take a vacation every year, perhaps even jetting off to exotic locations. If all goes according to plan, she'll get married, have babies in her twenties and thirties, send her kids off to university and then welcome her grandchildren in her sixties.

Take a closer look at that female fertility window. Those years are sandwiched in the middle of your busy life, your peak earning years, the time when you're exploring the world, busy buying cars and houses, doing everything you think you should do to create the lifestyle you desire. It doesn't look like such a long time now, does it?

And the truth is, despite all the media hype telling men they can get a woman pregnant at ninety, male fertility is finite too – it sharply declines after age forty.[4,5,6] Men often delay looking for help because they think it will be easy to get a woman pregnant and that, as a couple, they have 'plenty of time'. But again, if you've been trying for two years or more, it's highly unlikely that you're going to get pregnant by doing nothing, or worse, by simply continuing to do more of the same.

Many people put off starting a family until later in life because they assume it's better to spend crucial years making more money, buying more things, visiting more places – and that there will always be more time. But time is the one thing you can't buy. Of course, this isn't the case for everyone who seeks our help. Some people just haven't found the right partner until much later than they thought they would or decided to head down the solo reproduction road instead of waiting around but still didn't have success. And some have already been trying for years and have run out of ideas. It's a good thing you're reading this book right now, for if you take the right action, it may still be possible to give yourselves the best chance of creating the outcome you desire.

• TAKE A BREATH •

Grab a pen and mark your age on the 'Life in Months' map. Look at how many circles you have remaining in the fertility window. Think about all the things you want to do, be or have. Are you on track for fulfilling your ideal life? Are you taking charge of your highest priorities in life? Are you using your time and energy resources wisely?

With the right strategy and support, you may still have time to make a difference to your fertility window, but you must take charge and begin now.

References

1   Cooper, T.G., et al., World Health Organization reference values for human semen characteristics. *Human Reproduction Update*, 2010. 16(3).

2   Fisher, M.M., et al., What is in our environment that effects puberty? *Reprod Toxicol.*, 2014. 44.

3   Grindler, N.M., et al., Persistent organic pollutants and early menopause in U.S. women. *PLoS One*, 2015. 10(1).

4   Colasante, A., et al., The aging male: Relationship between male age, sperm quality and sperm DNA damage in an unselected population of 3124 men attending the fertility centre for the first time. *Archivio Italiano Di Urologia, Andrologia: Organo Ufficiale [di] Societa Italiana Di Ecografia Urologica E Nefrologica*, 2019. 90(4).

5   Emokpae, M.A., et al., Effect of senescence on some apoptosis and oxidative stress markers in infertile normozoospermic and oligospermic men: A cross-sectional study. *International Journal of Reproductive Biomedicine* (Yazd, Iran), 2018. 16(7).

6   Stone, B.A., et al., Age thresholds for changes in semen parameters in men. *Fertility and Sterility*, 2013. 100(4).

CHAPTER 2

It's About What You Choose To Focus On

'The trick in life is learning how to deal with it.'

Helen Mirren

Just about every day I wish I could snap my fingers and give my patients the baby they dream of. I also wish my magic finger-snapping could fix extreme poverty, world hunger, climate change and a host of global issues. But the magic doesn't lie in me. It lies in your taking charge of your circumstances and your choices. Watching back-to-back episodes of the latest TV series or bemoaning the state of the nation and your life isn't going to get you your baby.

There are things you can worry about (your areas of concern) and there are things you can do something about (your areas of influence). But you must choose wisely where you invest your energy because no matter how much you may dislike a particular weather pattern, for instance, you cannot control it. You can only influence your experience of it – by dressing appropriately, moving to another climate that pleases you more, and/or choosing your attitude. That's all. It's a choice. Becoming clear about what belongs in which area is of paramount importance when it comes to your long-term happiness.

TEST RESULTS
2-Week Wait
MISCARRIAGE
AGE
DELAYED TIME-TO-PREGNANCY
Social Expectations
"UNEXPLAINED" INFERTILITY
Suboptimal egg quality
GENETICS
SUBOPTIMAL SEMEN ANALYSIS
THYROID DISEASE
PCOS
Fibroids
Endometriosis

AREAS OF CONCERN

Where you live
WHAT YOU BUY
Where you work
WHAT YOU READ
RELATIONSHIPS
Exposure to Environmental Toxins
DIET & FLUID BALANCE
EXERCISE
MIND Stress
Epigenetics OVER MATTER
YOUR EMOTIONS AND EXPECTATIONS
SLEEP
Male and Female Reproductive Health
WHOLE BODY ALIGNMENT
Nutritional Supplementation

AREAS OF INFLUENCE

People often run the risk of spending too much of their time on areas of concern, worrying about the things they cannot change or control, such as how long it's taking for the test results to come back from the lab and how they'll feel if the results aren't what they would like to see. Time and energy spent on areas of concern is effort taken away from your areas of influence. By investing your time in your areas of influence, you can change the course of your life. What will you choose?

Taking charge of your choices – for as long as it takes – is the best way to be able to predict your future (in every area of your life).

Contrary to what you may have been taught, many things that contribute to your optimum fertility are, to a large extent, within your ability to influence – and while you can never control any outcome, you always have complete control over your input into any particular situation.

Underestimating or dismissing your ability to influence your results, coupled with a general apathy regarding educating yourself about how to take charge of your fertility journey, is what may well be keeping you infertile. There is much that's within your control, including your lifestyle choices.

That's the great news.

Your attitude to your fertility journey is also within your control. Ultimately, you and your partner are in charge as a unit, because fertility is a team sport. It's up to you, as a team, whether you'll choose to exercise the power that only you have to transform your results once and for all, or whether you'll continue going around in circles.

I'd like to share the story of a professor who stood in front of a class and placed rocks in a jar until it was full. He asked the class: 'Is this jar full?' The students replied yes. Then the professor added pebbles to the top of the jar and gently shook it until the pebbles filled the spaces between the rocks. 'What about now?' he asked. The students agreed that it was. The professor proceeded to add sand to the top of the jar until all the sand trickled down and nothing would move inside the jar, and then he added water to the brim. Only then did the professor concede that the jar was full.

In my version of this story, the rocks are one's health, relationships and resources. If nothing but the rocks were in the jar, you'd still have every opportunity to thrive. The pebbles represent other valued things (career, hobbies, creativity, etc) and the sand and water represents the 'small stuff' – the stuff that's typically fleeting or of little consequence in the grand scheme of things and your long-term happiness. If the sand and water were placed in the jar first, the pebbles and rocks simply wouldn't fit. The point I'm highlighting here is that it's important to connect with and prioritise what really matters. For this to occur, clarity on your current obstacles to optimum fertility, and most importantly how to effectively address them, is vital.

One of my Fertility Challenge™ participants once told me: 'You've taught me many valuable things, but the biggest learnings have been in relation to changing my mindset, setting behavioural goals and realising that I don't have to be a victim to infertility.' I did a happy dance at this realisation.

• TAKE A BREATH •

Draw your own areas of concern and influence diagram (in terms of your fertility). Where would you put your nutrition? Are you in control of what you eat? Will you choose to stop smoking? Drinking alcohol? Will you choose to exercise? Who is in ultimate control of your going to the gym?

Most people want a simple, magical answer to their fertility difficulties. They believe that if they go down the IVF or intracytoplasmic sperm injection (ICSI) route (despite being unhealthy), take a magic nutrient or herb, and do this 'massage and yoga thing', everything will be fine. This seemingly innocent approach is a dangerous trap. Amazonian monkey pee for breakfast, lunch and dinner isn't going to get you pregnant. Nor will, in practical terms, connecting with your spirit baby (but go for it if it makes you feel better).

I get it. You're lost and don't know who to trust. So, just in case any of it could be true, you end up doing a whole lot of disjointed and ineffective activities in the hope of realising your dream. This is what being misinformed, overwhelmed and confused looks like – leading to a huge waste of precious fertile time.

People try to take down the brick wall that lies between them and their dream one brick at a time. They pull off one brick and then try to squeeze through the crack. When they realise they'll never fit through, they move down the wall and pull off another random brick. The empty spaces quickly fill up with sadness, bitterness and an unwillingness to try anything that could actually help. But deep down, they know they're not done, so they keep at that wall, without the proper tools or strategy, sustaining further 'injuries' along the way.

The reality is that most couples have barely scratched the surface of what they could do to effectively overcome their fertility challenge, despite all the 'activities' (and the thousands of dollars wasted). It's vital to understand that when seemingly minor obstacles to health and fertility get compounded, they create something quite major. Ultimately, determining the best way to transform your results must be a deeply systematic and methodical process that takes the whole couple into consideration – not just parts of one person.

As I always tell my patients, removing a brick at a time from the infertility wall is ineffective, at best. Instead, you need a great big bulldozer to smash that wall down, clear the way and build a path to the healthy baby of your dreams. It's messy work in the beginning, but the results are infinitely more satisfactory in the medium to long term.

You have more power than you think. Forget about spending your time in those areas of concern. Dedicate yourself to your realm of influence, educate yourself so you know exactly what you need to do, and then, with the right support, knowing you're on the right path, take action until (not if) you have your outcome.

CHAPTER 3

Fertility Is Not
A Numbers Game

'True freedom is understanding that we have a choice
in who and what we allow to have power over us.'

Meryl Streep

Couples undergoing assisted reproductive treatments (ART) are
often told that success is a 'numbers game'. That the more they
do it, the greater the chances of success due to its 'luck of the draw'
nature. I believe that the 'numbers game' and 'luck of the draw'
approaches to fertility treatment threaten clinical equipoise, and in
many cases blur ethical boundaries.

A vast body of research validates every recommendation I share
in this book, so the question is: why isn't it shared with every fertility
patient worldwide before embarking on expensive and what could
be much more effective treatment?

The answer is sad and multifactorial, yet simple.

Most clinicians spend little time reading the scientific evidence
published in medical journals and updating their knowledge. As
well, there's an erroneous, intrinsic bias that technology is more
effective than the body's own innate wisdom and that it can 'fix'
everything. Of course, this isn't the case. My patients show this
to be true every day with their multiple failed IVF/ICSI cycles.
Finally, technological interventions for infertility have become a

multi-billion-dollar industry since their inception in 1978, with investors and stakeholders expecting a return on their investment. This return depends on more people doing more cycles.

I have strong reservations about this worrying trend happening around the world; women are being herded like cows towards repeated IVF and/or donor egg cycles before a couple has done the work to optimise their health to improve their fertility results (and they're often 'herded' under the guise of 'you're too old, your eggs are no good and we shouldn't waste any time').

I've lost count of how many hundreds of times our patients who've experienced multiple failed IVF cycles and are told these things then go on to conceive and deliver more than one healthy biological child – once we finally address the heart of the matter, in their specific situation, taking both prospective parents into serious consideration. And those who still need IVF, finally do take home a baby because we do the work of removing the obstacles to success prior to yet another attempt that would have otherwise been a futile exercise.

The big problem with thinking that assisted reproductive technology or treatments (ART) is a foolproof science is that it's not true. ART, which includes techniques such as in vitro fertilisation (IVF) and intracytoplasmic sperm injection (ICSI), is *not* a magic bullet and often still fails as a result of unresolved obstacles to optimum health and fertility. I'm impartial about what my patients need in order to eventually get pregnant and have a healthy baby – as long as the prescription is made after considered effort to understand the real cause of the problem (along with appropriate health promotion education), which is seldom solely someone's age or a single reproductive gamete. ART is a marvellous tool, and if after thorough assessment and treatment we believe a couple need ART in their specific circumstances, I'm the first to recommend it. But I know IVF/ICSI and even donor programs will just be a big waste of money if the issues that are getting in their way aren't appropriately addressed within an adequate time frame, in advance. I want the couples we treat to go through a procedure like IVF/ICSI with the best possible chance of it working the *first time*, rather than after the 'recommended' international guideline of three to five attempts.

For best results for you and your future child, it's essential that you don't buy into fear or your doctor's love of statistics. Or that you don't continue going through failed cycle after failed cycle because this is a 'numbers game' or the 'luck of the draw'. ART is a miracle of modern technology and a wonderful adjunct to treatment where necessary. But, I have a fundamental issue with this type of 'losing strategy', where couples are advised to just 'keep on keeping on' with minimal focus on what can be improved or optimised in between cycles to yield better patient experiences and results – particularly since current scientific evidence points to an increased risk of rare cancers (and potentially other conditions) in IVF/ICSI-conceived children and their mothers.[1,2,3,4]

I believe couples, even if for no other reason than successful continuation of the species, need and deserve much better education regarding all the issues that can hinder their chances of getting and staying pregnant – before embarking upon ART. A collaborative, educational approach to fertility treatment is urgently needed for the sake of public health worldwide. And through my experience treating thousands of couples, when an integrative approach is implemented effectively, it has the positive side effect of keeping patients engaged, and in addition, further improving overall treatment success rates. As a result, this type of partnership is a win-win for all concerned.

Currently, most patients undergoing ART are simply advised to keep trying – without any further recommendation regarding what they can do to improve their chances of success. Most people for whom treatment isn't working will at some point hear that treatment hasn't worked because of poor egg quality, at which point donor eggs or embryos will likely be recommended. But what couples hardly ever hear is that while it's the egg's responsibility to address and correct DNA errors within the sperm, if those male cells aren't the healthiest they can possibly be, the egg must use even more of its own internal resources (and mitochondrial energy, closely linked to its viability and eventual embryonic development) to correct sperm issues.[5,6] As a result, the chances of fertilisation and early embryonic development are often arrested.[7,8] And so the couple continue going around in circles on the fertility journey while the male is continually (and wrongly) told that ejaculating in a cup is the limit of his contribution to a couple's chances of taking home a healthy baby.

Additionally, a woman's body goes through a major upheaval throughout a fertility treatment cycle; it's pounded with chemicals and toxins. And it's not only the body that suffers. Most people's mental health takes a beating. Their finances are depleted and their overall quality of life is diminished while the clock continues ticking.

Given that, as much as we try, we still can't hack biology, it makes no sense to embark on ART if both partners aren't in the best possible shape they could be – especially when there is evidence of previously failed attempts or long-standing infertility or recurrent miscarriage. Without a better strategy, in these cases couples unfortunately just keep on having more of the same lack of results. Ultimately, the time will pass anyway, but if you're putting in the effort to become the healthiest version of yourself along the way, you're adding rather than withdrawing from your health and fertility 'bank account'.

Unfortunately, most people want a simple answer to their fertility issues. They hope that a complex history can be summarised and solved in 'three simple steps', or that a baby will materialise with a magic remedy and minimal effort.

The truth is that if you've tried many different things and still don't have the result you're looking for, your current team is likely missing some pieces of your fertility puzzle. Perhaps the very pieces that are required to transform your results.

Some couples will never conceive without IVF, and this is a fact; but ignoring obstacles to optimum health and fertility and thinking certain issues can be bypassed by technology is never a good idea – especially when ART is necessary. If you want the most direct route to baby, even if it feels like the long, slow and drawn-out one, I assure you, from decades of clinical experience, as in the rabbit and the turtle fable, you must address all of the relevant impediments to your healthiest possible self before applying technology if you want to fundamentally transform your results.

Let's look at the minor factors – the multiple, often seemingly small and irrelevant obstacles to optimum health and fertility – and why they're so important.

References

1   Pontesilli, M., et al., Subfertility and assisted reproduction techniques are associated with poorer cardiometabolic profiles in childhood. *Reproductive Biomedicine Online*, 2015. 30(3).

2   Reigstad, M.M., et al., Cancer risk in women treated with fertility drugs according to parity status – A registry-based cohort study. *Cancer Epidemiology Biomarkers & Prevention*, 2017. 26(6).

3   Spector, L.G., et al., Association of in vitro fertilization with childhood cancer in the United States. *JAMA Pediatrics*, 2019.

4   Sullivan-Pyke, C.S., et al., In vitro fertilization and adverse obstetric and perinatal outcomes. *Seminars in Perinatology*, 2017. 41(6).

5   Meseguer, M., et al., Effect of sperm DNA fragmentation on pregnancy outcome depends on oocyte quality. *Fertility and Sterility*, 2011. 95(1).

6   Tamburrino, L., et al., Mechanisms and clinical correlates of sperm DNA damage. *Asian Journal of Andrology*, 2012. 14(1).

7   Alvarez Sedó, C., et al., Effect of sperm DNA fragmentation on embryo development: Clinical and biological aspects. *JBRA Assisted Reproduction*, 2017. 21(4).

8   Colaco, S., et al., Paternal factors contributing to embryo quality. *Journal of Assisted Reproduction and Genetics*, 2018. 35(11).

CHAPTER 4

The Minor Things To Major In

'Courage is the most important of all the virtues
because without courage, you can't practice
any other virtue consistently.'

Maya Angelou

When it comes to infertility, most people look for the *big* reason (or reasons) their ultimate result keeps eluding them. Newsflash: it's the minor factors that are getting in your way and stopping you from getting pregnant. These minor factors are the very bricks that make up the 'wall of infertility'. They are the 'little' subclinical issues your clinician often fails to point out when they gloss over a semen analysis report or a couple of pages of blood test results to categorically pronounce 'it all looks fine'. Meanwhile, you're still not pregnant. The big problem with these categorical pronouncements is that in nine out of ten cases, they don't address the issues that ultimately mean the difference between having a baby or not.

Sometimes you might even know about these issues but you're told, 'It's nothing major, just keep trying', or you're given the usual – no advice and a referral to IVF.

Again, those little, seemingly inconsequential issues or results that the practitioner treating you dismisses may in fact mean infinitely more than initially meets the eye. If the team in charge of your treatment doesn't take the time to understand all the pieces of your giant fertility puzzle, the important pieces will remain stuck in some box at the back of some metaphorical cupboard somewhere. And you'll be forever lost in an ineffective strategy that leads to no baby.

I cannot count the number of times I've heard my patients relay horror stories about the people treating them. One of my patients, who is now blessed with her own little miracle (we did everything we needed to help her change her situation), was once told by her 'specialist' that if she wasn't an 'old hag' she would be pregnant by now. She was only thirty-six at the time. Another patient told me, with tears in her eyes, that she'd been 'branded' with the following charming words: 'This is what happens to women like you who don't see the ticking pendulum of the fertility clock of doom.' As if any woman should have to endure such treatment.

When all is said and done, fertility boils down to the little things – as is confirmed by epidemiological studies around the globe. In his bestselling book *Getting Pregnant*, illustrious, late Professor Robert Jansen describes the fertility model he used for many years and that continues to be applied today to explain the 'statistics' of the fertility world. Table 1.1 shows the effect of multiple minor abnormalities on monthly fertility and on the likely time needed to get pregnant.[1]

Table 1.1

Number of Factors	Average Monthly Fertility (%)	% Pregnant in 2 Years	% Pregnant in 3 Years	Average Time Needed to Get Pregnant
0	20	93.6	96.7	3 Months
1	5	63.6	75.5	2 Years
2	1	20.7	28.9	7 Years
3	0.2	4.7	6.9	40 Years

I want to point out that as much as I like this statistical analysis as a thought-provoking, educational model to guide understanding about this concept, I don't believe any of my patients is a number, and I often speak about the fact that the numbers (age, laboratory results and years of infertility) do not define them or what's actually possible in their situation. What's important is clarity regarding the so-called minor factors. There's absolutely no doubt in my mind that when it comes to fertility, minor abnormalities spell out the difference between having a baby and never becoming a parent.

What are the numbers in Table 1.1 telling us? At peak fertility, on average, a couple has a 20% chance of conception in any given month and an average time to pregnancy of three months. Add one minor factor to the mix and the chances of conception fall to 5% and the average time to pregnancy increases to two years. Two minor factors and a couple's chance of pregnancy plummets to 1% and the average time to pregnancy increases to seven years. Adding just one more minor factor brings a couple's total to only three minor factors, but all of a sudden, their chances of conception fall to 0.2% and the average time to pregnancy is an impossible forty years!

Italian economist Vilfredo Pareto (1848–1923) had it right when he said that for many events, roughly 80% of the desired effect comes from 20% of the causes. Not all minor factors are made equal, and when it comes to my patients (and most people who wish to overcome long-standing infertility and recurrent miscarriage), I'm convinced that knowing what minor factors we're dealing with is only the beginning. The real results come from understanding what 20% effort will deliver 80% of our results – and continuing this application until a couple is holding their healthy baby in their arms.

So, what are these minor abnormalities causing major heartache?

Perhaps the sperm isn't shaped how it should be, or a man doesn't have as much sperm as would be ideal, or the sperm's swimming ability is compromised. Maybe your partner likes a drink or thinks regular visits to a fast-food joint are part of a 'balanced' diet, and as a result, his sperm is affected by excessive oxidation and its DNA becomes highly fragmented – put simply, it's not as healthy as it could be – thus placing an extra (and in some cases, fatal) burden on the amount of work an egg needs to do in order to support fertilisation and proper embryonic development.

Perhaps you're still smoking or have a few kilos to lose. Here's a classic scenario: you're a confessed chocoholic and, due to polycystic ovarian syndrome, you're carrying excess weight or have insulin resistance, leading to erratic ovulation caused by other ensuing hormonal imbalances. Add a history of sexually transmitted infections (STIs) or a thyroid that's not working as effectively as it could be (an already classic presentation with PCOS). Or maybe you've been diagnosed with endometriosis, or your ovarian reserve is diminished for whatever reason.

Taken individually, these 'little things' aren't the sole reason you're not yet pregnant, but when added together, they comprise a considerable issue.

It's not unusual in our thorough investigations to find that a couple has more (and sometimes way more) than fifteen minor abnormalities impacting their optimum fertility. These seemingly inconsequential anomalies are not dismissed in our clinic because we understand categorically that when minor factors are combined, their effects are compounded – dramatically decreasing a couple's chances of getting pregnant and taking home a healthy baby. These minor abnormalities are of extraordinary consequence for a couple trying to conceive. Especially when the couple has been trying to get pregnant for over two years, has experienced miscarriage or has gone through failed ART cycles. To me, these clues signal the need to start afresh with a systematic, methodical, holistic and integrative approach such as the F.E.R.T.I.L.E. Method®.

One patient told me, 'There were things that I didn't know I didn't know. But also, there were things that I really haven't been walking the talk on that I kind of knew. You've pushed me to stick to everything that I know I need to do, and it has helped me to stop panicking just because I'm forty-one. Knowing that there's so much my partner and I can now do towards making our dream come true – this understanding has given me hope.' This couple ended up delivering a beautiful, healthy baby girl.

Not knowing what you don't know about the minor factors and, more importantly, not knowing how to best address them are the top reasons you're not yet pregnant or holding the baby of your dreams in your arms.

Dramatically improving your odds of success on your fertility journey can come down to making a concerted effort on a mere 20% of compounding factors. But figuring out which are the 20%, where to start and what to focus on in your particular situation is more than half of the work required to transform your results.

I can guarantee that if you're reading this book and you're not yet pregnant despite all you've tried, the impediments to fertility discussed here apply to you. If you want a baby as quickly as possible, I urge you to become proactive and begin thinking in terms of minor factors. If you've been diagnosed with 'unexplained infertility' (that is, your doctor said 'everything looks normal, just keep trying'), it's absolutely time to rethink your strategy. I've seen so many couples waste precious years not understanding that they could have changed their results much sooner.

• TAKE A BREATH •

To help you understand the current and specific impediments to your optimum fertility, I've created the free Fertility Quiz which you can access online. This quiz allows you to answer six key questions to give you further clarity on the next steps you can take to overcome infertility and miscarriage, even when other treatments have failed. Take the free Fertility Quiz here: http://thefertile.me/freeassessment

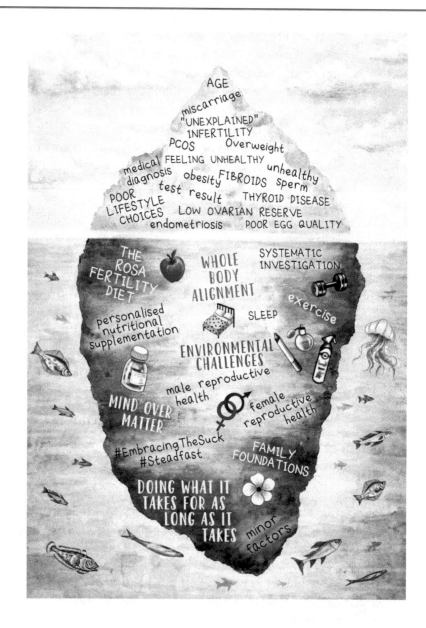

In the next section, I'm going to show you how to begin taking charge of the factors you can most easily and directly influence to optimise your fertility over the next 120 days and beyond – factors such as your diet, lifestyle and mindset, fertility toxins in your home, and more. These helpful tactics are part of a much more comprehensive treatment plan that can make an enormous difference to couples who wish to overcome infertility and miscarriage.

Minor factors are real, and the F.E.R.T.I.L.E. Method®, which I developed over the last couple of decades and which underpins our effective treatments and diagnostic processes, ensures you achieve, not only clarity about the obstacles which must be removed from your path to help you achieve parenthood but also provides a practical and definitive path to help you achieve just that.

Again, the choice is yours. Continue doing what you've been doing or get clear about what you need to know in order to revolutionise your results once and for all, utilising the necessary strategies required in your specific situation to create your healthy baby.

Just as minor factors compound to create seemingly impossible odds, small, incremental and consistent improvement and a bucketload of commitment and courage compound to create the ultimate foundation for success in any endeavour – especially this one. So, keep the faith, do what it takes and enjoy the ride. Your life is the masterpiece that only *you* can create.

References

1 Jansen, R., *Getting Pregnant: A Compassionate Resource to Overcoming Infertility and Avoiding Miscarriage.* 2nd ed. 2003, Crows Nest, Australia: Allen & Unwin.

CHAPTER 5

The Top Seven
Fertility Misconceptions

'A goal without a plan is just a wish.'

Antoine de Saint-Exupéry

I've spent two decades educating couples on the things they need to know regarding fertility, and seven misconceptions continue to make their rounds in the fertility world. I'd like to set the record straight, here and now.

Fertility misconception 1: Your eggs are past their used-by date if you're over thirty-five

This blanket statement is untrue. Statistically speaking, as women age fertility levels do decline over time, but remember, most women in the general population aren't as educated as they could be about fertility, or doing the best they can to optimise it.

Many of our patients are over forty when they conceive and take home their babies, as you'll read about in some case studies later. Why? Because we look at fertility as a team sport. If the egg is struggling for any reason, having the best-quality sperm possible is paramount. We help couples optimise their chances together, instead of blaming an arbitrary age or singular focus, such as the egg, when natural conception is hindered. In this way, we are to a certain extent able to mitigate the impact of the side effects of ageing. By addressing these side effects, we can positively influence egg quality. A great amount of emerging scientific research also confirms this finding.[1,2] We may still not be able to increase a woman's ovarian reserve (the number of eggs you're born with) through the application of technology; however, the scientific research is clear about the fact that egg quality is not immutable.[3,4] Addressing the underlying causes of why the egg isn't as healthy as it could be – perhaps due to excessive oxidation,[5,6,7] lack of nutrients,[8,9,10] too many toxins, [11,12] and much more – is a better, more holistic approach to help couples create their ultimate outcome. Of course, not every person is going to conceive, irrespective of their age.

While you cannot increase your ovarian reserve (the number of eggs you're born with), given the scientific knowledge we have today, we know it's absolutely possible to improve egg quality.[13,14,15,16,17,18,19,20] And this is something we focus on with clear drive in my clinic. There are many ways to improve egg quality, which I'll share later.

The bottom line is that it's not true that if you're over thirty-five, you categorically don't have good-quality eggs that are able to produce a healthy baby. It's still possible for you to conceive and carry a healthy baby to term – and you will most definitely have to work for it. The latter is a fact.

Fertility misconception 2: ART is the only option

In some cases, ART (IVF, ICSI, etc) is necessary, but it should always be the last resort, not the first, second or third step. A couple who undergoes any form of reproductive treatment without the appropriate preparation and proper focus on minor factors will often walk away disappointed, heartbroken and financially drained.

Tracey will share her story later in the book. She experienced multiple failed IVF cycles (over a ten-year period of trying to conceive) before coming to me; she felt our treatment was her last resort. After three and a half months on our program, she fell pregnant naturally. She was forty and her husband was fifty.[21]

Fertility misconception 3: Miscarriage and implantation failure are just 'luck of the draw'

Most medical systems around the world don't view it as necessary to investigate miscarriages before a couple has experienced a minimum of three. I've never experienced a miscarriage, but just the thought of having to experience *three* before something is done about it is devastating. I've successfully treated a large number of women who have been through the ordeal of recurrent miscarriage, and the trauma they know is beyond devastating – especially from the point of eight weeks' gestation onwards.

So in my clinic, our approach isn't to wait and 'hope' for the best. Instead, we take a proactive approach towards our patients' fertility treatment, especially as it relates to the prevention of miscarriage and implantation failure. We screen for issues we can easily pre-empt because there are common causes that can positively influence if a person is properly assessed and treated as part of a holistic, integrative and proactive approach. This is at a minimum a compassionate, ethical and professionally effective approach to treating the patients who have already gone through so much on their fertility journey. In our clinic, we specialise in treating difficult and complex cases; there are often many concomitant factors which when unknown or left unaddressed will delay pregnancy even further, if not indefinitely, for many couples. We typically work with patients who have experienced recurrent miscarriage and/or infertility for over two years, and who have tried many different treatments and therapies without the success they'd hoped.

As a result, we go back to systematically and methodically ruling out the possible causes of miscarriage that are well established in the scientific literature, adding to our investigations and treatment protocols accordingly, as more is discovered in these areas.

Through years of research and deliberate observation regarding this topic, at this time we have identified and work from the paradigm of nine major categories or 'umbrella' reasons for miscarriage. (Of course, it's not possible to totally reduce a couple's miscarriage risk or implantation failure to just one of the nine categories – there are always a combination of factors at play in any one circumstance.) In each of these categories there are a few to as many as a dozen factors – and we're constantly finding and adding pieces to these puzzles, compiling comprehensive lists that can guide and help speed up our investigative process for our patients. What is certain is that many of these factors, both in isolation and in combination, may impact an embryo's ability to implant into the uterine lining and effectively develop into a healthy baby.[22,23]

Nine major factors that may lead to miscarriage

1. **Endocrinological:** These are hormonal factors, reproductive as well as metabolic hormone deficiencies and/or imbalances, such as diabetes and thyroid disorder.[24,25] Many metabolic disorders will impact the ability to conceive – detailed investigations are required depending on each patient's specific clues and symptomatology.

2. **Anatomical:** These are specifically related to problems such as fibroids, placenta abruption, umbilical cord issues and haemorrhage before or during labour that cause miscarriage or late miscarriage/stillbirth.[26,27,28,29] In alignment with my F.E.R.T.I.L.E. Method®, in the first stage of our treatment, the preconception preparation, we ensure fibroids are specifically addressed (where necessary and possible) through surgical intervention prior to conception attempts recommencing to increase a couple's chances of taking home a healthy baby.

3. **Uterine defects:** Such defects may include congenital uterine abnormalities, which will require surgical intervention (in addition

to our treatment), for example septate and bicornate uterus or acquired conditions such as cervical insufficiency.[30,31] The traditional approach to treating cervical insufficiency is via cervical cerclage[32,33] and progesterone pessaries.[34,35] Although this is a diagnosis possible only during pregnancy, it's useful to be aware of it as a possible causative factor. If you've experienced miscarriage, be sure to broach the topic with your doctors for proper diagnosis sooner rather than later during a new pregnancy.

4. **Infections:** Many infections which negatively impact the chances of taking a healthy pregnancy to term are asymptomatic.[36] STIs are known causes of infertility and miscarriage, and lesser-known systemic infections can also play a harmful role.[37,38,39] Other infections to rule out and/or treat in the preconception stage and beyond include Lyme disease, toxoplasmosis, listeriosis, ureaplasma, mycoplasma, cytomegalovirus and more. Maintaining a healthy immune system in general is vital because even a particularly severe case of the flu can negatively affect a pregnancy, which is not simply and easily fixed with flu vaccine.

5. **Immunological:** Various types of miscarriage antibodies and alloimmune and autoimmune conditions will increase the risk of miscarriage and implantation failure.[40,41,42,43] We have a special interest in our clinic in the immunological factors impacting fertility and focus heavily on this area to ensure nothing is left to chance.

6. **Genetic:** Parental abnormalities may need to be ruled out or better understood. Genetic testing for both partners is recommended in the investigative stage of a comprehensive fertility treatment protocol. For instance, a mutation in the MTHFR gene may play a role in extended time to pregnancy and miscarriage recurrence. This mutation affects approximately half of the world's population; it impairs the body's ability to create a biologically active form of folate: methylfolate. The biochemical impairment caused by this

genetic mutation negatively impacts DNA regulation, immunity, and neurotransmitter and hormone production as well as the body's ability to properly detoxify. The resultant inability to effectively process all B vitamins, especially folate, can also lead to severe birth defects in the developing embryo and foetus, in addition to increasing the risk of miscarriage, infertility, preeclampsia, cardiovascular disease and more.[44,45] MTHFR mutation will also negatively impact the maturation of the egg and sperm, so it must be ruled out in both prospective parents (among other predisposing genetic mutations).[46,47,48] Despite the fact that MTHFR mutation has been made incredibly popular in recent years, it is important to note that if you think it is all about a MTHFR mutation you are missing the point. There are many gene variants, which must be assessed and, if found, addressed in order to decrease the risk of implantation failure and miscarriage, as a part of a holistic and integrative treatment approach.

7. **Male factor:** 50% of miscarriages occur due to poor sperm quality (low motility, poor morphology and/or high levels of DNA fragmentation).[49,50,51] When sperm is clinically or subclinically impaired (aka average or just *below* average, despite it being fine to use through IVF or worse, ICSI) the rate of implantation failure and miscarriage risk increases; remember, fertility is a team sport – without quality sperm, the egg must utilise more of its own resources to sustain the necessary exponential cellular division of an embryo post-fertilisation. And the negative impact of poor-quality sperm (despite the available high-tech solutions) doesn't only stop couples from having a baby naturally – failed IVF and ICSI are also much more likely. A large meta-analysis, which included 8,068 treatment cycles, concluded that male factor has a 'negative effect on clinical pregnancy following IVF and/or ICSI treatment'.[52]

If the egg quality is compromised or a couple is dealing with a low ovarian reserve, then the sperm must ideally be well above average in quality for best results. A man's contribution to a healthy baby is infinitely more remarkable than most IVF specialists will have you believe. It can be the ultimate difference between a couple being able to create a healthy baby or not.[53,54]

8. **Reproductive toxicants:** This is a major public health concern that remains inadequately addressed. Dangerous and toxic chemicals are currently accepted by a major portion of Western society (completely erroneously) as safe. A lack of education and public awareness coupled with inadequate policy to safeguard and protect our global community means that health and fertility are continuously under attack as a result of exposure to these toxins. There is conclusive scientific evidence that daily exposure to chemicals commonly available on the shelves of supermarkets (and which enter most households and workplaces) is highly detrimental to optimum health and reproductive outcomes. This very real (chemical) threat to a couple's ability to conceive and take a healthy pregnancy to term is highly underestimated.[55,56,57] These toxicants come in various disguises. They're found in the form of cleaning products, make-up and personal-care items, pest control and more – marketed widely, as the panacea for modern life, and camouflaged by beautiful colours and dangerous fragrances (perfumes should be labelled 'pure-fumes'). All of these different chemicals have one thing in common: they directly and indirectly negatively impact general, and specifically reproductive, health.[58,59] These compounds, as well as those found in plastics of every kind (including the 'BPA-free' ones, which are full of other equally dangerous but less publicised bisphenols, plasticisers and other toxic chemicals),[60,61,62] pesticides,[63,64,65] heavy metals (lead, mercury, arsenic),[66,67,68] 'antibacterial agents',[69,70] organic solvents (industrial pollutants

that make their way into the home through new furniture and furnishings, as well as cleaning products, etc),[71,72,73,74] cigarette smoke (active and passive),[75,76,77,78,79,80,81,82] alcohol,[83,84,85,86] and so much more, are persistent environmental and, in some cases, occupational chemical hazards couples get exposed to daily. This exposure is detrimental to the egg as well as to the sperm structure and function, and negatively affects the quality and health of developing embryos, foetuses and infants.[58-86] Many couples don't even get to the point where they see a positive pregnancy test because, unfortunately, the developing embryo is so sensitive to these exposures that post-fertilisation development (if it occurs at all) stops before a positive result (or very shortly after). What's really sad is that so many miscarriages and foetal abnormalities and malformations could be avoided if people were properly educated about these dangerous chemicals and how best to avoid them.

9. **Idiopathic or unexplained:** The problem with any unexplained diagnosis is that it's simply too easy to fall back on. A thorough assessment of a patient's case is always required, with as many minor factors as possible identified for prospective treatment before some generic *unexplained* label may even potentially be entertained. I'll admit that there are factors which negatively impact a couple's chances of conceiving and keeping a healthy pregnancy to term that haven't been fully studied, remain incompletely understood, or perhaps haven't yet been discovered. However, let's also be honest about the fact that just like every reason for conception failure is not a case for donor egg, not every case of implantation failure or recurrent miscarriage is 'unexplained' – a couple is thoroughly, systematically and methodically investigated at the outset of treatment (and ongoing as necessary), to uncover and further correlate relevant minor

factors in their specific case, as the very first recommended step of the F.E.R.T.I.L.E. Method®.

Before seeing me, one of my patients had eight miscarriages. Her husband had a triple sperm defect (low count, poor morphology and motility – and this was a few short years back when DNA fragmentation tests for sperm weren't yet commercialised; had they been, I'm sure we would have found abnormalities there also). They were conceiving but unable to take a healthy pregnancy to term. Through our thorough investigations, we discovered, among many other minor factors, that the mercury levels in her blood were forty times higher than the maximum toxicity range acceptable in humans. Mercury is a toxicant directly linked to infertility and miscarriage. We worked with this couple, taking a multifaceted approach that incorporated medically administered chelation therapy to remove the high levels of mercury from her system while addressing all the other minor factors. It took twelve months to get this patient's mercury levels down allowing for the (mandatory) four-month break post-chelation therapy before she could start trying to conceive again. But the results quite literally speak for themselves – they now have four beautiful children.

This is what I dream of, pray for and work hard to help all my patients create. I don't like to leave anything to chance; I want to cover all bases – at least all the known ones. And I like to have plans A, B, C, D, E, F and G clearly outlined at the beginning of a couple's treatment so we know where we're headed (always course-correcting as new information comes to the fore). I run my clinic and my life based on Kaizen – the Japanese principle of constant improvement. It's impossible at the beginning of a couple's treatment to know everything we need to know to help them create a healthy baby. We must keep searching and applying intelligence, knowledge, experience and curiosity to every situation until we discover enough to help our patients create their ultimate outcome. We'll never be perfect, but perfection is overrated anyway. I'd rather get started and course-correct as necessary than wait for some idealistic and impossible version of perfection in any endeavour, and I teach my patients to do the same. Frankly, life – and one's reproductive window – is too short to continue doing more of the same, while expecting a different result. We put on our detective goggles and, in a focused, committed and methodical way, work hard to find the necessary puzzle pieces that complete the picture we are working towards. That's why we get results when 'everything else has failed'. The key is to stay focused *until* (you get your result) rather than *if* (you get your result). As one of my mentors recently reminded me, 'The only place success comes before work is in the dictionary.'

Fertility misconception 4:
Just relax and you'll get pregnant

If you're anything like my patients, this myth will grate on you. You've probably heard this hundreds of times by now, and at some point you may even have believed it and started stressing about stressing.

Of course, stress does play a role in our inability to conceive and keep a pregnancy to term. Our bodies still very much work like they did 10,000 years ago, when a human's sole aim was survival (which involved running away from the sabre-toothed tiger). When our stress levels are high, the body will suppress the functions of organs and systems not necessary for warding off immediate danger. I cover this in detail in Prescription 8: Understanding The Numbers Behind Your Test Results.

It's important to dampen the body's stress response if it's getting out of control. Relaxation, meditation and mindfulness are all important. But you now understand that the compounding effect of minor (and maybe even some major) factors make up the wall that stands between you and the baby you hope to create. If overcoming infertility (and miscarriage) was as simple as relaxing, every single person who's ever been on a holiday would get pregnant.

Fertility misconception 5: Low AMH requires egg donation or IVF

My patients have taught me that just because you have low AMH, it doesn't categorically mean you can conceive only through egg donation or ART.

Later, you'll hear from Jenny. After twenty (fully stimulated) rounds of IVF, four years of trying to conceive, and being told by several doctors that there was nothing further that could be done and egg donation was their only hope, she and her husband put in the necessary effort and determined action and conceived naturally (when Jenny was thirty-nine). How did this happen? We addressed all their minor factors. Being proactive, we neutralised the effects of the things we couldn't change and worked on everything we could *until* they got their outcome.

Fertility misconception 6: Infertility is a woman's issue

Saying that infertility and miscarriage is a woman's issue is the same as saying synchronised swimming is a solo sport. Need I say more? It's time we fully recognise and properly understand the importance of the male contribution to a couple's chances of taking home a healthy baby.

Fertility misconception 7: Nothing can be done for male infertility other than IVF or ICSI

Appropriately understanding why a man has been diagnosed with infertility rather than just accepting a poor semen analysis result at face value is critical if you want to overcome and conquer this challenge.

Sperm is highly susceptible to damage from chemicals, radiation, heat, junk food, alcohol, smoking, recreational substances and more. Our patients prove every day just how much improving their lifestyle and removing obstacles to optimum health can help to optimise sperm quality.

Even in some cases of Klinefelter syndrome or Y chromosome microdeletions, if any sperm is present, it may be possible to optimise its quality for better results through ART. I've also been told by my patients who haven't been able to achieve enough improvement for a cycle with a man's own sperm how much happier they were in knowing they'd done everything they possibly could before choosing donor sperm. Doing the work to improve their general and sperm health irrespective of the immediate outcome gave them invaluable peace of mind and a sense of no regrets regarding their fertility journey and whatever other choices they could make on their journey to parenthood. What my patients have also demonstrated and taught me over the last two decades is that knowing you've done your best and have learned from the experience along the way helps you create a healthier, and therefore happier, family foundation. This pre-work into creating a family is what this whole exercise is about in the first place. No one wants a baby for the sake of a baby – we want love, connection, belonging: family. The solid foundations required to create a well-adjusted child within a family unit (however that looks for each generation) are laid right from within this very experience along the fertility journey and beyond – not in spite of it.

Table 2.1

Contributing factors to male infertility[87,88,89]

1. Abnormal sperm parameters – poor sperm morphology, motility or count, lowered semen volume, increased DNA fragmentation, presence of sperm antibodies

1. Anatomical problems – varicocele, seminal tract obstruction, testicular damage due to radiation, trauma, torsion and/or cyst

2. Congenital anomalies – systemic and/or urogenital tract eg hypospadias, cryptorchidism, etc

3. Genetic defects – autosomal aberrations, CTFR mutation, sex chromosome abnormalities, Y chromosome microdeletions

4. Hormonal imbalances – hypogonadism, hypothalamic, hypopituitarism, etc

5. Infections and STIs

6. Lifestyle risk factors – cigarette smoking, alcohol intake, use of illicit drugs, anabolic steroids and other medications, obesity, psychological stress, diet, caffeine intake, elevated scrotal temperatures

7. Oncological diseases

8. Sexual dysfunctions – anorgasmia, anejaculation, retrograde ejaculation

References

1   Mihalas, B.P., et al., Molecular mechanisms responsible for increased vulnerability of the ageing oocyte to oxidative damage. *Oxidative Medicine and Cellular Longevity*, 2017.

2   Vollenhoven, B., et al., Ovarian ageing and the impact on female fertility. *F1000Research*, 2018. 7.

3   Chang, Y., et al., Egg quality and pregnancy outcome in young infertile women with diminished ovarian reserve. *Medical Science Monitor: International Medical Journal of Experimental and Clinical Research*, 2018. 24.

4   Dumesic, D.A., et al., Oocyte environment: Follicular fluid and cumulus cells are critical for oocyte health. *Fertility and Sterility*, 2015. 103(2).

5   Almeida, C.P., et al., Clinical correlation of apoptosis in human granulosa cells – A review. *Cell Biology International*, 2018. 42(10).

6   Guan, Y., et al., Cell-free DNA induced apoptosis of granulosa cells by oxidative stress. *Clinica Chimica Acta; International Journal of Clinical Chemistry*, 2017. 473.

7   Lu, J., et al., A novel and compact review on the role of oxidative stress in female reproduction. *Reproductive Biology and Endocrinology: RB&E*, 2018. 16.

8   Gaskins, A.J., et al., Dietary patterns and outcomes of assisted reproduction. *American Journal of Obstetrics and Gynecology*, 2019.

9   Gu, L., et al., Metabolic control of oocyte development: Linking maternal nutrition and reproductive outcomes. *Cellular and Molecular Life Sciences: CMLS*, 2015. 72(2).

10 Jahangirifar, M., et al., Dietary patterns and the outcomes of assisted reproductive techniques in women with primary infertility: A prospective cohort study. *International Journal of Fertility & Sterility*, 2019. 12(4).

11 Hipwell, A.E., et al., Exposure to non-persistent chemicals in consumer products and fecundability: a systematic review. *Human Reproduction Update*, 2019. 25(1).

12 Petro, E.M.L., et al., Endocrine-disrupting chemicals in human follicular fluid impair in vitro oocyte developmental competence. *Human Reproduction* (Oxford, England), 2012. 27(4).

13 Kasum, M., et al., The role of female obesity on in vitro fertilization outcomes. *Gynecological Endocrinology: The Official Journal of the International Society of Gynecological Endocrinology*, 2018. 34(3).

14 Kitano, Y., et al., Oral administration of l-carnitine improves the clinical outcome of fertility in patients with IVF treatment. *Gynecological Endocrinology: The Official Journal of the International Society of Gynecological Endocrinology*, 2018. 34(8).

15 Machtinger, R., et al., Association between preconception maternal beverage intake and in vitro fertilization outcomes. *Fertility and Sterility*, 2017. 108(6).

16 Ruebel, M.L., et al., Obesity leads to distinct metabolomic signatures in the follicular fluid of women undergoing in vitro fertilization. *American Journal of Physiology. Endocrinology and Metabolism*, 2019.

17 Souter, I., et al., The association of protein intake (amount and type) with ovarian antral follicle counts among infertile women: Results from the EARTH prospective study cohort. *BJOG: an international journal of obstetrics and gynaecology*, 2017. 124(10).

18 Xu, Y., et al., Pretreatment with coenzyme Q10 improves ovarian response and embryo quality in low-prognosis young women with decreased ovarian reserve: A randomized controlled trial. *Reproductive Biology and Endocrinology: RB&E*, 2018. 16(1).

19 Zhang, T., et al., Di(2-ethylhexyl)phthalate: Adverse effects on folliculogenesis that cannot be neglected. *Environmental and Molecular Mutagenesis*, 2016. 57(8).

20 Zheng, X., et al., Inositol supplement improves clinical pregnancy rate in infertile women undergoing ovulation induction for ICSI or IVF-ET. *Medicine*, 2017. 96(49).

21 Rosa, G., video creation story: 'We conceived naturally after 10 years of infertility and previously failed IVF'.

22 Bashiri, A., et al., Recurrent implantation failure – update overview on etiology, diagnosis, treatment and future directions. *Reproductive Biology and Endocrinology: RB&E*, 2018. 16(1).

23 Jauniaux, E., et al., Pathophysiology of histological changes in early pregnancy loss. *Placenta*, 2005. 26(2–3).

24 Matjila, M.J., et al., Medical conditions associated with recurrent miscarriage – Is BMI the tip of the iceberg? *European Journal of Obstetrics, Gynecology, and Reproductive Biology*, 2017. 214.

25 Zhang, Y., et al., Patients with subclinical hypothyroidism before 20 weeks of pregnancy have a higher risk of miscarriage: A systematic review and meta-analysis. *PLoS One*, 2017. 12(4).

26 Baumfeld, Y., et al., Placenta associated pregnancy complications in pregnancies complicated with placenta previa. *Taiwanese Journal of Obstetrics & Gynecology*, 2017. 56(3).

27 Haruyama, R., et al., Causes and risk factors for singleton stillbirth in Japan: Analysis of a nationwide perinatal database, 2013–2014. *Scientific Reports*, 2018. 8(1).

28 Ravishankar, S., et al., Placental findings in feto-maternal hemorrhage in livebirth and stillbirth. *Pathology, Research and Practice*, 2017. 213(4).

29   Wang, X., et al., The impact of noncavity-distorting intramural fibroids on the efficacy of in vitro fertilization-embryo transfer: An updated meta-analysis. *BioMed Research International*, 2018.

30   Cakmak, H., et al., Implantation failure: Molecular mechanisms and clinical treatment. *Human Reproduction Update*, 2011. 17(2).

31   Neveu, M.-E., et al., Fertility and pregnancy outcomes after transvaginal cervico-isthmic cerclage. *European Journal of Obstetrics, Gynecology, and Reproductive Biology*, 2017. 218.

32   Liddiard, A., et al., Elective and emergency cervical cerclage and immediate pregnancy outcomes: A retrospective observational study. *JRSM short reports*, 2011. 2(11).

33   Wafi, A., et al., Influence of cervical cerclage interventions upon the incidence of neonatal death: A retrospective study comparing prophylactic versus rescue cerclages. *Facts, Views & Vision in ObGyn*, 2018. 10(1).

34   Alfirevic, Z., et al., Vaginal progesterone, cerclage or cervical pessary for preventing preterm birth in asymptomatic singleton pregnant women with a history of preterm birth and a sonographic short cervix. *Ultrasound in Obstetrics & Gynecology: The Official Journal of the International Society of Ultrasound in Obstetrics and Gynecology*, 2013. 41(2).

35   Karbasian, N., et al., Combined treatment with cervical pessary and vaginal progesterone for the prevention of preterm birth: A randomized clinical trial. *The Journal of Obstetrics and Gynaecology Research*, 2016. 42(12).

36   Kuon, R.J., et al., Higher prevalence of colonization with Gardnerella vaginalis and gram-negative anaerobes in patients with recurrent miscarriage and elevated peripheral natural killer cells. *Journal of Reproductive Immunology*, 2017. 120.

37   Schuppe, H.-C., et al., Urogenital infection as a risk factor for male infertility. *Deutsches Ärzteblatt International*, 2017. 114(19).

38   Tao, X., et al., Relationships between female infertility and female genital infections and pelvic inflammatory disease: A population-based nested controlled study. *Clinics*, 2018. 73.

39   Tsevat, D.G., et al., Sexually transmitted diseases and infertility. *American Journal of Obstetrics and Gynecology*, 2017. 216(1).

40   Lédée, N., et al., The uterine immune profile may help women with repeated unexplained embryo implantation failure after in vitro fertilization. *American Journal of Reproductive Immunology* (New York, N.Y.: 1989), 2016. 75(3).

41   Miko, E., et al., Characteristics of peripheral blood NK and NKT-like cells in euthyroid and subclinical hypothyroid women with thyroid autoimmunity experiencing reproductive failure. *Journal of Reproductive Immunology*, 2017. 124.

42   Promberger, R., et al., A retrospective study on the association between thyroid autoantibodies with β2-glycoprotein and cardiolipin antibodies in recurrent miscarriage. *Iranian Journal of Allergy, Asthma, and Immunology*, 2017. 16(1).

43   Santos, T.d.S., et al., Antiphospholipid syndrome and recurrent miscarriage: A systematic review and meta-analysis. *Journal of Reproductive Immunology*, 2017. 123.

44   Turgal, M., et al., Methylenetetrahydrofolate reductase polymorphisms and pregnancy outcome. *Geburtshilfe Und Frauenheilkunde*, 2018. 78(9).

45   Zhang, Y., et al., The association between maternal methylenetetrahydrofolate reductase C677T and A1298C polymorphism and birth defects and adverse pregnancy outcomes. *Prenatal Diagnosis*, 2018.

46   Cornet, D., et al., Association between the MTHFR-C677T isoform and structure of sperm DNA. *Journal of Assisted Reproduction and Genetics*, 2017. 34(10).

47   Gong, M., et al., MTHFR 677C>T polymorphism increases the male infertility risk: A meta-analysis involving 26 studies. *PLoS One*, 2015. 10(3).

48   Shahrokhi, S.Z., et al., The relationship between the MTHFR C677T genotypes to serum anti-müllerian hormone concentrations and in vitro fertilization/intracytoplasmic sperm injection outcome. *Clinical Laboratory*, 2017. 63(5).

49   Jayasena, C.N., et al., Reduced testicular steroidogenesis and increased semen oxidative stress in male partners as novel markers of recurrent miscarriage. *Clinical Chemistry*, 2019. 65(1).

50   Kamkar, N., et al., The relationship between sperm DNA fragmentation, free radicals and antioxidant capacity with idiopathic repeated pregnancy loss. *Reproductive Biology*, 2018. 18(4).

51   Robinson, L., et al., The effect of sperm DNA fragmentation on miscarriage rates: A systematic review and meta-analysis. *Human Reproduction* (Oxford, England), 2012. 27(10).

52   Simon, L., et al., A systematic review and meta-analysis to determine the effect of sperm DNA damage on in vitro fertilization and intracytoplasmic sperm injection outcome. *Asian Journal of Andrology*, 2017. 19(1).

53   Anawalt, B.D., Approach to male infertility and induction of spermatogenesis. *The Journal of Clinical Endocrinology and Metabolism*, 2013. 98(9).

54   Piccolomini, M.M., et al., How general semen quality influences the blastocyst formation rate: Analysis of 4205 IVF cycles. *JBRA Assisted Reproduction*, 2018. 22(2).

55   Kumar, S., Occupational, environmental and lifestyle factors associated with spontaneous abortion. *Reproductive Sciences* (Thousand Oaks, Calif.), 2011. 18(10).

56   Martinez, R.M., et al., Urinary concentrations of phenols and phthalate metabolites reflect extracellular vesicle microRNA expression in follicular fluid. *Environment International*, 2019. 123.

57   Smarr, M.M., et al., Preconception seminal plasma concentrations of endocrine disrupting chemicals in relation to semen quality parameters among male partners planning for pregnancy. *Environmental Research*, 2018. 167.

58   Darbre, P.D., Overview of air pollution and endocrine disorders. *International Journal of General Medicine*, 2018. 11.

59   Rudel, R.A., et al., Endocrine disrupting chemicals in indoor and outdoor air. *Atmospheric Environment* (Oxford, England: 1994), 2009. 43(1).

60   Ejaredar, M., et al., Phthalate exposure and childrens neurodevelopment: A systematic review. *Environmental Research*, 2015. 142.

61   Philips, E.M., et al., Effects of early exposure to phthalates and bisphenols on cardiometabolic outcomes in pregnancy and childhood. *Reproductive Toxicology* (Elmsford, N.Y.), 2017. 68.

62   Rochester, J.R., et al., Bisphenol S and F: A systematic review and comparison of the hormonal activity of Bisphenol A substitutes. *Environmental Health Perspectives*, 2015. 123(7).

63   Chiu, Y.-H., et al., Association between pesticide residue intake from consumption of fruits and vegetables and pregnancy outcomes among women undergoing infertility treatment with assisted reproductive technology. *JAMA Internal Medicine*, 2018. 178(1).

64   Frazier, L.M., Reproductive disorders associated with pesticide exposure. *Journal of Agromedicine*, 2007. 12(1).

65   Martenies, S.E., et al., Environmental and occupational pesticide exposure and human sperm parameters: A systematic review. *Toxicology*, 2013. 307.

66   Buck Louis, G.M., et al., Heavy metals and couple fecundity, the LIFE Study. *Chemosphere*, 2012. 87(11).

67   Quansah, R., et al., Association of arsenic with adverse pregnancy outcomes/infant mortality: A systematic review and meta-analysis. *Environmental Health Perspectives*, 2015. 123(5).

68   Vejrup, K., et al., Prenatal mercury exposure, maternal seafood consumption and associations with child language at five years. *Environment International*, 2018. 110.

69   Smarr, M.M., et al., Male urinary biomarkers of antimicrobial exposure and bi-directional associations with semen quality parameters. *Reproductive Toxicology* (Elmsford, N.Y.), 2018. 77.

70   Wang, X., et al., Maternal urinary triclosan concentration in relation to maternal and neonatal thyroid hormone levels: A prospective study. *Environmental Health Perspectives*, 2017. 125(6).

71   Conforti, A., et al., Air pollution and female fertility: A systematic review of literature. *Reproductive Biology and Endocrinology: RB&E*, 2018. 16(1).

72   Cowell, W.J., et al., Prenatal exposure to polybrominated diphenyl ethers and child attention problems at 3–7 years. *Neurotoxicology and Teratology*, 2015. 52(Pt B).

73   Le Cornet, C., et al., Parental occupational exposure to organic solvents and testicular germ cell tumors in their offspring: NORDTEST study. *Environmental Health Perspectives*, 2017. 125(6).

74   Snijder, C.A., et al., Occupational exposure to chemical substances and time to pregnancy: A systematic review. *Human Reproduction Update*, 2012. 18(3).

75   Burke, H., et al., Prenatal and passive smoke exposure and incidence of asthma and wheeze: Systematic review and meta-analysis. *Pediatrics*, 2012. 129(4).

76   Dechanet, C., et al., Effects of cigarette smoking on reproduction. *Human Reproduction Update*, 2011. 17(1).

77   Hyland, A., et al., Associations between lifetime tobacco exposure with infertility and age at natural menopause: The Women's Health Initiative Observational Study. *Tobacco Control*, 2016. 25(6).

78   Lee, S.L., et al., Foetal exposure to maternal passive smoking is associated with childhood asthma, allergic rhinitis, and eczema. *The Scientific World Journal*, 2012.

79   Li, J., et al., Effect of exposure to second-hand smoke from husbands on biochemical hyperandrogenism, metabolic syndrome and conception rates in women with polycystic ovary syndrome undergoing ovulation induction. *Human Reproduction* (Oxford, England), 2018. 33(4).

80   Neal, M.S., et al., Sidestream smoking is equally as damaging as mainstream smoking on IVF outcomes. *Human Reproduction* (Oxford, England), 2005. 20(9).

81   Sharma, R., et al., Cigarette smoking and semen quality: A new meta-analysis examining the effect of the 2010 World Health Organization laboratory methods for the examination of human semen. *European Urology*, 2016. 70(4).

82   Zhang, R.-P., et al., The effects of maternal cigarette smoking on pregnancy outcomes using assisted reproduction technologies: An updated meta-analysis. *Journal of Gynecology Obstetrics and Human Reproduction*, 2018. 47(9).

83   Aboulmaouahib, S., et al., Impact of alcohol and cigarette smoking consumption in male fertility potential: Looks at lipid peroxidation, enzymatic antioxidant activities and sperm DNA damage. *Andrologia*, 2018. 50(3).

84   Dodge, L.E., et al., Women's alcohol consumption and cumulative incidence of live birth following in vitro fertilization. *Journal of Assisted Reproduction and Genetics*, 2017. 34(7).

85   Fan, D., et al., Female alcohol consumption and fecundability: A systematic review and dose-response meta-analysis. *Scientific Reports*, 2017. 7.

86   Rossi, B.V., et al., Effect of alcohol consumption on in vitro fertilization. *Obstetrics and Gynecology*, 2011. 117(1).

87   Durairajanayagam, D., Lifestyle causes of male infertility. *Arab Journal of Urology*, 2018. 16(1).

88   Leaver, R.B., Male infertility: An overview of causes and treatment options. *British Journal of Nursing*, 2016. 25(18).

89   Punab, M., et al., Causes of male infertility: A 9-year prospective monocentre study on 1737 patients with reduced total sperm counts. *Human Reproduction* (Oxford, England), 2017. 32(1).

CHAPTER 6

The Five Critical Mistakes That Hold You Back

'The price of inaction is far greater than
the cost of making a mistake.'

Meister Eckhart

Before we look at what you can do to take charge of your fertility results, let's look at some mistakes that hold people back. I once did a survey of my patients regarding what critical mistakes they wish they could have been warned about before they made them and received about 1,000 responses. These were people who had been trying to conceive and take home a healthy baby for several years and had many failed treatments under their belt.

There were some clear trends, which I've condensed and categorised – in the end, it all boiled down to five critical mistakes. These appear here in no particular order because in my experience, these mistakes are relevant for different people at different times (although they're all made at some point once a person has been on this journey long enough).

It's important to also acknowledge that while these critical mistakes are common to many couples, everyone's emotional, physical and spiritual experience of the journey is different.

These five mistakes are always underpinned by multiple *minor factors* that are often completely overlooked.

Critical mistake 1: Stressing about stressing

Not surprisingly, this is one of the biggest issues. By stressing, we decrease our chances of conception because physiological response mechanisms – fight, flight or freeze – are hardwired into our DNA for survival.

There's a clear need to manage the stress of the fertility journey, as well as the impact it may have on a couple's relationship. There are both positive and very negative ways to cope with the heightened stress couples experience during this period in their lives. For example, some choose alcohol and/or cigarettes as a momentary decompressing mechanism. Unfortunately, this kind of strategy also keeps couples infertile. When working to overcome infertility and miscarriage, it's vital to choose your decompressing mechanisms wisely.

Let's say that smoking is your form of stress relief.[1,2] Smoking (actively or passively) has been shown to negatively impact each stage of male and female reproduction, as well as embryonic development. It decreases a woman's fertile reproductive life by up to five years, bringing on early menopause, and it drastically decreases a man's ability to make sperm and increases his risk of testicular failure – not to mention that IVF is much more likely to fail for smokers than for their non-smoking counterparts, regardless of other minor factors. Similarly, if you or your partner's stress release is alcohol, you, as a couple, will substantially decrease your chances of conception and increase your risk of implantation failure and miscarriage. Although safety guidelines have been adjusted over the years, there is no real safe alcohol-consumption and smoking limit when it comes to getting pregnant and taking home a healthy baby. Each of these toxicants has similar negative effects on the quality of the egg and sperm.

Effectively managing stress is vital in terms of optimum fertility. In Part 2, I'm going to show you how you can do that, and how you can put stress back in your area of influence.

Critical mistake 2: Forgetting that fertility is a team sport

It's a huge mistake to exclude men from the fertility journey. Too few fertility treatment options support men appropriately or take into account how they're feeling, their stress levels, and what they're doing to improve their health. Particularly early on in their journey, couples rarely understand how mission-critical it is for both partners to engage and do their best to optimise their chances of taking home a healthy baby. Heck, most men don't even get asked to have blood tests as a part of their fertility workup. But the worst case is when, as I've seen in my own clinic (numerous times), a couple has experienced more than two years of infertility or repeated miscarriages and, up until we start working together, has never even had a semen analysis. It's important to remember that a semen analysis (like any other result) is a snapshot of a moment in time – biology is constantly changing based on immediate and long-term exposures. Even a severe case of the flu can wipe out quality sperm for months on end,[3,4,5] and infections are only one 'tiny' minor factor. Keep a finger on the pulse, so to speak, when monitoring fertility over time. If your partner's sperm was fine six, twelve or seventy-two months ago, it doesn't mean it's fine today.

It's utterly ludicrous that men are often left to the side of the fertility equation – they're 50% of said equation. And even if we were to slice it up differently and say (as it's often said) that 40% of infertility is due to female factor, 40% to male factor and 20% to an unexplained/idiopathic combination, they still contribute to 50% of that 20%. In my experience, men want to contribute and do their part once they're educated about the absolute importance of their role. Men want to be part of the solution (and if you are a man reading this book, you've just proved it. Kudos, I salute you). Men often feel helpless on the fertility journey precisely because they'd like to be able to help and don't know how. Typically, health caregivers ensure the male stays disconnected from the process through lack of education, as well as through excessive focus placed on the woman's 'issues'. The man becomes a detached spectator of the whole process, rather than an active and valuable participant who can add immense (physical and emotional) value to the entire process.

As well, men typically have a strong need to understand detail and see proven information. They don't want to simply be told what to do and what to believe. Don't get me wrong – women can be like this too. But if men aren't engaged from the beginning, they often disconnect from the process altogether. This is why our approach is different. We want to ensure both partners are engaged and working together as a team, so we focus first on the vital education that helps couples understand the *why* and *how*, to support action and to develop realistic expectations around outcomes. Engaging both partners, enhancing communication and improving the way partners work together, as a team, on this journey is critical to its long-term success. My patients tell us that this approach also helps further consolidate the solid foundation every family needs, and for this I'm grateful.

Critical mistake 3: Lack of knowledge

The number one reason couples become stuck on their fertility journey is that they 'don't know what they don't know'.

If you're reading this book, it's likely you're experiencing the 'I don't know what I don't know' syndrome. When couples come to me and say, 'We've tried *everything*, and nothing has worked.' I reply, 'You haven't fully implemented the F.E.R.T.I.L.E. Method® yet, so you haven't yet tried everything.' The reason they're saying this is because they've hit the limits of their metaphorical ceiling of knowledge. And as Albert Einstein said, 'We cannot solve our problems with the same thinking we used when we created them.'

To solve problems we must grow; we must push through our limitations with purpose, certainty and self-belief, always asking better questions: 'How else?' 'Who else?' 'What else?' Sometimes you may need a break to catch your breath and refocus, but only you can decide when and where to stop and pursue a different path. And this is why I love the Japanese principle of Kaizen (constant improvement) so much. If you aren't constantly improving, you hit a wall and stay there, banging your head against it. My other favourite method for problem solving is to call for reinforcements. This is the time to summon the metaphorical bulldozer, clear the path, reimagine it and then build it – from beginning to baby.

For me, calling reinforcements involves finding a guide or a mentor: someone who has created what I want and/or has a proven track record in helping others do so. I hire them to Sherpa me up that mountain.

For couples on the fertility journey, there's a lack of knowledge on so many levels, from simply not knowing what questions to ask to not knowing how best to proceed or to whom to turn for help. Sadly, over the years, I've witnessed this mistake cost people a reasonable chance of having a baby altogether. People who, had they been proactive, could have had a very different result. People who chose to do the bare minimum and remained complacent in terms of taking charge of their fertility (while telling themselves they were doing 'everything'), but ultimately deep down thinking someone else would rescue them and not making it their business to educate themselves on what was required to transform their results. Those who are most unaware think that even though they're not getting pregnant, they have their bases covered and are already doing 'all the right things' because they're already doing all they had been recommended or are taking supplements, eating well, exercising and trying to manage their stress. They fail to understand that it's just not enough to do what everyone else who's getting the result they want does (I'll address this in the breakout feature titled 'Epigenetics and the heroin addict syndrome'); they fail to realise they're wasting precious time they'll never get back. Now is the time for action based on proven, effective knowledge. This book is a good start – but on its own, it may not be enough for many couples.

Those who complete our comprehensive couple fertility and health appraisal – a fifty-plus-page document designed to help our team understand exactly what areas aren't working – a pivotal part of the F.E.R.T.I.L.E. Diagnostic Assessment™ we make available, will gain the precise understanding they need about what specifically isn't working in their fertility situation and, through the Natural Fertility Breakthrough Program™, what they need to do about it. This is a highly customised and personalised strategy that takes a couple's entire situation into consideration (as well as a personalised path for individuals undergoing solo reproduction). By the time someone has gone through this entire process with our clinic, they understand what's getting in the way of their results, specifically what their minor factors are and what to do about them. People also discover what they don't know, and this is typically why they come to us – they want to get to the root cause of the issue and have it addressed as directly as possible. They also learn that we must address the body's needs from within the limitation of its biological frameworks. We cannot change the fact that biologically, it takes an egg eight months to mature, or the fact that major improvements to sperm parameters often take two or three sperm cycles to fully develop.[6,7] Still, there is much that can be done in a relatively short time frame to transform a couple's entire situation – given the right strategy. Keep reading.

Critical mistake 4: Wasted resources

Plenty of people waste their time continuing to do the same thing over and over, for years, without a result and carry on thinking that it will all turn out okay. Remember Albert Einstein's wisdom? Don't waste your time. Almost 50% of everyone surveyed talked about the time, money and heartache invested to date, without results, saying, 'If only I'd known there was another way.'

Later you'll read about one of our couples who experienced over twenty failed IVF cycles, to the tune of about $10,000 to $15,000 per cycle. That amounts to a deposit on a very nice house by the sea.

After undertaking the Natural Fertility Breakthrough Program™, they ended up conceiving naturally.

It's about taking the right action and doing whatever it takes that makes the difference. The key is not to delay. Don't waste any more time, money or heartache.

Critical mistake 5: Regret

The final mistake those surveyed spoke of is regret – the regret of not giving it their all, of not taking charge of their situation and making their own choices, of allowing decisions to be made for them. Many survey respondents said they regret rushing into IVF only to discover it wasn't the only option, or that there were things that needed to be or could have been done to improve their chances of IVF success (before thousands of dollars were wasted).

Again, I have nothing against ART. To the contrary, I see it as a godsend technology for some couples who would never have been able to conceive otherwise, and we support many couples through their IVF/ICSI journey. The issue I have is that assisted reproductive techniques in general are treated as the silver bullet that will 'fix the problem' with minimum effort, rather than a useful tool to aid nature where absolutely necessary – once a couple's minor factors are comprehensively and effectively addressed.

There are no shortcuts

There is no way around this fact. We work to ensure that every couple we serve can one day look back on their fertility journey and know that they've done their best – that if it didn't happen, for whatever reason, it wasn't because they didn't put in the work or the effort. This way, they can journey on without regret. Above all, though, we want to ensure they see considerable improvement in their quality of life as a result of holistic treatment, irrespective of the outcome.

Your best may be different from day to day, but as long as you give it your all, wherever you choose to draw the line in terms of having a baby, you'll never have any regrets. Some will pursue the objective of having a baby only if they can conceive naturally. Some will consider IVF/ICSI. Some will choose donor egg, donor sperm, donor embryo, surrogacy or even adoption. Those who will truly do everything, do so because their outcome is a baby – no matter how that little being arrives in their lives. The key is to know that you've left no stone unturned when it comes to your heart's contentment.

I know the difference the steps I share in this book (and beyond) can make for a couple who's been struggling to create their family dream. This is why I decided, decades ago, to dedicate my life to making real change for people on this journey. Revolutionising the way couples are cared for is only the beginning. There is so much power in taking charge, in doing what it takes, in finding your strength, and I want that difference in people's lives to be my legacy. Change can only come from doing what it takes. If you want me and my team on your side, holding your hand from beginning to baby, read on.

• TAKE A BREATH •

Take a moment to think about the mistakes you may be making on your fertility journey. Are you fully informed? Are you and your partner on the same page? Have you reached a compromise on how far you're both willing to go? Are you taking charge of your daily choices and consciously making them rather than allowing inertia to take over your life and dictate how things will turn out?

Choosing to take charge, educate yourself, become fully conscious of all the choices you can make in any given circumstance and work in alignment with your partner, for the highest good of all concerned, is my favourite strategy for dramatically decreasing stress and increasing quality of life.[12,13,14]

No more regrets, no turning back

'We must all suffer from one of two pains: the pain of discipline or the pain of regret. The difference is discipline weighs ounces while regret weighs tons.'

Jim Rohn

In a series of six scientific studies summarised in the paper titled *The ideal road not taken: The self-discrepancies involved in people's most enduring regrets*,[8] researchers identified three elements that make up a person's sense of self.

1. Your 'actual' self consists of qualities that you believe you possess.

2. Your 'ideal' self is made up of the qualities you want to have (hopes, goals, aspirations or wishes); these make up your most fulfilled self.

3. Your 'ought' self is the person you feel you should be, according to duties, responsibilities, social norms and agreements (typically in search of external validation).

When asked to name their single biggest regret in life, 76% of the participants in the six studies said it was not fulfilling their ideal self. People are quicker to take steps to live up to their duties and responsibilities, all those things they 'ought' to do, than they are to live up to their own goals and aspirations. The study's lead investigators hypothesised that people's most enduring regrets in life come from discrepancies between their actual and ideal selves.

The type of person you become depends on the actions you take and the choices you make daily. The right habits, developed early, are key to an ideal life. It's vital to act on your hopes and desires so you can live this ideal life rather than place an over-idealistic 'hope' in where inertia will take you. In my experience, while some begrudge

71

making disciplined efforts in the short-term, inaction is what people regret long term. So, stop making excuses for yourself and your partner now. You'll never regret taking charge of your life and taking positive action towards creating your ideal outcomes.

• TAKE A BREATH •

Remember the buck stops with you. Completely irrespective of anyone else or anything outside of yourself, on your deathbed, what will you regret? What type of person will you have been? Will you have taken action to live a fulfilled life? Your ideal life? Will you have taken charge of your challenges and worked until you conquered them?

In Parts 2 and 3 of this book, I'm going to show you how, by taking responsibility for your daily choices, in as little as six months (that's only six circles on the 'Life in Months' map), you'll be in an infinitely better position to live your best life – now. We'll look at creating the best version of yourself (physically and emotionally) as a way to optimise health and fertility and build the best foundation for a happy and healthy family life. All of your 11 Pillars of Fertility Foundations™ areas must be in alignment if you truly want to experience the breakthrough you deserve.

As Martin Luther King Jr said, 'Faith is taking the first step even when you don't see the whole staircase.' Results ultimately come from taking a whole lot of little steps, one after the other, after the other. Eventually, they'll lead you to the miracle of looking into your baby's eyes for the first time – no matter how they came to you.

So, what are you waiting for?

'[It's about] how many times you stand up, and are brave and you keep on going.'

Lady Gaga

I once heard a joke that stayed with me as a deep truth. I like to tell it to my patients, but since I'm a hopeless joke teller, I made it into more of a story. For me, it sums up the folly of waiting for the right sign or the right moment.

As the 'story' goes, a guy was stuck on his rooftop in a flood, praying to God for help. A man in a rowboat came by and shouted to the guy on the roof, 'Jump in, I can save you.'

The stranded guy shouted back, 'No, it's OK, I believe in God and I know he's going to save me.'

So the rowboat went on by.

Then a motorboat came by and the fellow in the motorboat shouted, 'Jump in, I can save you.'

The stranded guy replied, 'No thanks, I know God will save me. I have faith.'

So the motorboat went on by.

By this time, the stranded guy was holding on to pieces of floating debris.

Then a helicopter came by and the pilot shouted down, 'Grab this rope and I'll lift you to safety.'

The stranded guy once again replied, 'It's OK, I have faith. I know God will save me.'

So the helicopter flew away.

Soon, the man could no longer remain afloat, and he drowned and died. In Heaven, he got his chance to discuss this whole sorry situation with God. 'I had faith in you, but you didn't save me!' he said. 'I don't understand why!'

God replied, 'I sent you a rowboat, a motorboat and a helicopter. What more did you expect?'

I'm a firm believer in 'thy will be done' but not over and above 'do your part and the Heavens will come to your aid'. Remaining separate from your ideal outcomes in life under the guise of 'God knows what he's doing' is a massive cop-out as far as I'm concerned. By handing over full responsibility for your life to your god or fate, knowing full well you have choices and free will, is akin to picking up a 1,000-piece puzzle and expecting it will just solve itself. A less than winning strategy.

I've found that men take a particularly laid-back approach when it comes to their own and their partner's fertility. Perhaps it's because they're less attached to the outcome of having a baby; or they want to be the rock in the relationship and don't want to cause their partner undue stress; or they don't fully understand fertility or the fact that difficulties conceiving aren't static and that with the right approach, infertility and miscarriage risk are changeable. Whatever the reason, 'waiting and seeing' doesn't get you a baby. Especially because a woman's fertility is categorically finite. After menopause, a woman can no longer conceive without a donor egg (if her partner's sperm is still in reasonable shape – which isn't the case for many men over forty-five) or a donor embryo.[9,10,11]

If you really need a sign, take this book as one and let's get to work.

• TAKE A BREATH •

What are you waiting for? What's stopping you from taking action to create the very best version of yourself now?

In Part 2, I'll introduce you to the 11 Pillars of Fertility Foundations™, lead you through nine fertility recommendations I share with participants in my online, educational event The Fertility Challenge™, and explain the F.E.R.T.I.L.E. Method® – the basis for all my effective fertility programs and education.

References

1   Buchmann, A.F., et al., Cigarette craving increases after a psychosocial stress test and is related to cortisol stress response but not to dependence scores in daily smokers. *Journal of Psychopharmacology* (Oxford, England), 2010. 24(2).

2   Childs, E., et al., Effects of acute psychosocial stress on cigarette craving and smoking. *Nicotine & Tobacco Research*, 2010. 12(4).

3   Dejucq, N., et al., Viruses in the mammalian male genital tract and their effects on the reproductive system. *Microbiology and Molecular Biology Reviews: MMBR*, 2001. 65(2).

4   Fraczek, M., et al., Mechanisms of the harmful effects of bacterial semen infection on ejaculated human spermatozoa: Potential inflammatory markers in semen. *Folia Histochemica Et Cytobiologica*, 2015. 53(3).

5   Salam, A.P., et al., The breadth of viruses in human semen. *Emerging Infectious Diseases*, 2017. 23(11).

6   McGee, E.A., et al., Initial and cyclic recruitment of ovarian follicles. *Endocrine Reviews*, 2000. 21(2).

7   Wu, H., et al., Preconception urinary phthalate concentrations and sperm DNA methylation profiles among men undergoing IVF treatment: A cross-sectional study. *Human Reproduction* (Oxford, England), 2017. 32(11).

8   Davidai, S., et al., The ideal road not taken: The self-discrepancies involved in people's most enduring regrets. *Emotion*, 2018. 18(3).

9   Almeida, S., et al., Fertility and sperm quality in the aging male. *Current Pharmaceutical Design*, 2017. 23(30).

10   Alshahrani, S., et al., Infertile men older than 40 years are at higher risk of sperm DNA damage. *Reproductive Biology and Endocrinology: RB&E*, 2014. 12.

11   Jenkins, T.G., et al., Sperm epigenetics and aging. *Translational Andrology and Urology*, 2018. 7(Suppl 3).

12   Duckworth, A., *Grit: The Power of Passion and Perseverance.* 2016, London, UK: Simon and Schuster.

13   Duckworth, A., et al., Self-Control and grit: Related but separable determinants of success. *Current Directions in Psychological Science*, 2014. 23(5).

14   Hammond, D.A., Grit: An important characteristic in learners. *Currents in Pharmacy Teaching & Learning*, 2017. 9(1).

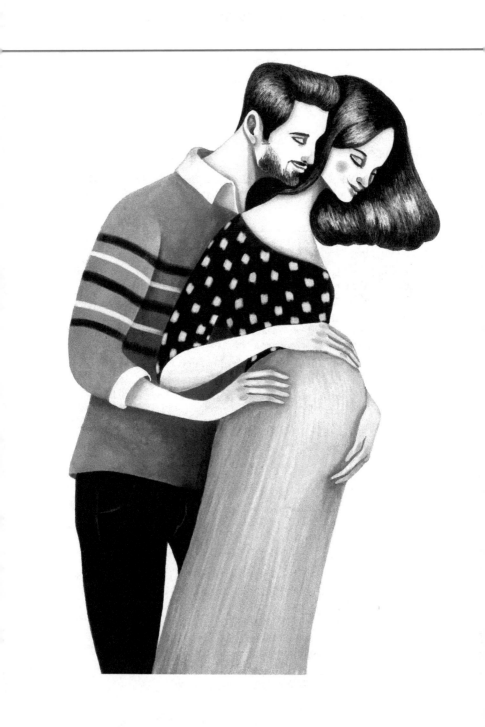

PART 2

FROM CHALLENGE TO BREAKTHROUGH

'Education is education. We should learn everything
and then choose which path to follow.
Education is neither Eastern nor Western, it is human.'

Malala Yousafzai

We hold our patients' hands from beginning to baby. As a result of our team's vast experience and formal qualifications in naturopathic and reproductive medicine, as well as in human genetics, we can blend the best of science and self-care for the benefit of our patients. We're ambitious in our goals for every couple we're honoured to serve. Each of our team members invests their individual time, talent and unmatched passion and care, wholeheartedly. I speak for the whole team when I say we want a baby for our patients as much as they want this outcome for themselves.

Why? Sure, our patients' babies are a testament to the success our world-class service helps couples achieve, overcoming infertility and miscarriage, even when other treatments have failed.[1] But there's more to it than that. Call me delusional, but I have this little (or major, if you prefer) idea that because of what we do, we make the world a better place. My team and I are fully invested in the idea that every healthy prospective parent who consciously works to overcome infertility and miscarriage and create a healthy baby – who then grows up into a healthy and happy adult – indeed makes the world a better place.

I've been practising and sharing the knowledge I'm about to share with you since I began learning it, in 1998. In 2001, I fully unleashed my passion when I began working in private practice and the Natural Fertility Breakthrough Program™ was born. Then, in 2010/2011, I launched The Fertility Challenge™. At the time, it was a little platform I'd created to educate my local community. Now, it's grown to have worldwide appeal. At the time of publishing the first edition of this book (2019), my team and I have taken more than 100,000 people from over 100 countries through our various programs. And over the years, we've seen more babies than I can count born to couples who were previously 'infertile' or who experienced recurrent miscarriage. In 2018, I created an Instagram account (@gabrielarosafertility) to feature some of the babies we know about and have permission to add to our gallery, and to feature the stories of many of the people we are privileged to serve. These are stories of courage, strength and determination.

This work has become a part of me over the years, and it's difficult to distinguish myself from it and everything that flourishes from it. I feel incredibly blessed and honoured to be able to serve at ever-growing levels. And now I'm here to guide you through the highly enlightening and positively life-transforming journey to optimum health and fertility. My wish is that this message spreads like wildfire for the benefit of millions of people worldwide – because optimum health (of which fertility is the ultimate derivative) is a finite resource, and without it, nothing else matters.

A small note of caution: although the information in this book is highly effective and, if applied appropriately and consistently, can be the answer to many people's problems, do not delay in seeking qualified, expert advice on your fertility situation. The number one concern I have when people tell me that they're doing some of my basic programs for the third, fourth or fifth time is that they're clearly missing large pieces of their fertility puzzle and time is passing.

Please don't let this be you. If you're proactively working through your situation with a qualified team utilising a complete and holistic strategy that incorporates the correct blend of science and self-care to create your outcome, that's a different situation. It requires time, as is the case for our patients on the Natural Fertility Breakthrough Program™. But trying to piece that fertility puzzle together yourself, or with minimally qualified support, is not a winning strategy, and you may be wasting precious time.

If you'd like our team to assess your situation so you can understand more about the issues affecting your specific fertility situation and how to address them, reach out to our team or participate in an obligation-free, complimentary Natural Fertility Breakthrough Program™ fertility assessment and information session. You can register here: http://thefertile.me/NFBPInfoSession. Your participation in one of these information sessions requires some important pre-work, so our team can best understand your fertility situation and determine if we can be of assistance in your specific case. Unless you're embarking on solo reproduction, you and your partner must participate together in the online information session to ensure you get the most out it – because fertility is a team sport.

Now, let's turn our attention to the breakthrough at hand. The aim is to get you into the best physical and mental shape before your next conception attempt. Remember, the quality of your egg today is determined by a lifetime of habits, and especially everything you've done in the last eight months (the amount of time it takes the female egg to mature, while sperm may take a little less). It's not possible to 'hack' biology. The body needs time to register and benefit from the changes you make, beginning now. My challenge to you is to implement one of my nine prescriptions I'll be making for you each day, taking the actions prescribed. Your willingness to take charge and 'get stuff done' (#GSD) is a prerequisite to working with my team. Above all, what we want to know is that you and your partner are fully committed to transforming your results and your journey.

CHAPTER 7

Start At The Beginning

'Kid, you'll move mountains! Today is your day!
Your mountain is waiting. So get on your way!'

Dr Seuss, *Oh, The Places You'll Go!*

We must start at the beginning. I'm here, ready and willing, to guide your discovery as well as support, encourage and inspire your commitment. And I expect you to be equally ready and willing to take charge of your fertility, your life and your results. I cannot do this for you. This matching of energies, working together as a team, is the only way our relationship can work to produce your ultimate outcome of a healthy baby. Everything you'll learn here will be transformational if you diligently and consistently *implement* this knowledge.

Put aside age, infertility, sperm abnormalities, medical complications, miscarriage, failed IVF cycles, etc. No matter what your unique situation is today, thousands have undertaken the forthcoming challenges and shared stories of how they've changed their lives for the better, once they fully committed and #GSD. Of course, there are always people who go through life looking to find fault and to prove how nothing works for them and how unfair it all is. People who quit before they even start. Those are not my people.

My first challenge to you is this: **Be the opposite of that person.** Dig deep and find your strength. I promise you there is incredible value in applying and mastering the basics and due process. Don't just quickly read the prescriptions, nodding and agreeing (or disagreeing because you haven't done your own research).

Here's an easy example. To lose weight, you need to burn more calories than you consume, or consume fewer calories than you burn – it's a simple equation. Eating well and exercising sufficiently is the only way to truly and concretely realise the goal of being at your ideal weight, despite so much hype on this topic. Intellectually, you know that you 'should' get yourself to a healthy weight (or whatever other goal you may need to achieve in your specific situation) to optimise your egg quality or sperm parameters, but be honest – are you actually doing what you know will help you? Determinedly, daily, *consistently*?

Look at it another way. Just because you don't believe eating right and going to the gym every day for a couple of years will deliver you a bikini body doesn't mean the strategy is flawed and that it hasn't worked for millions of people before you. It just means you've chosen not to take charge and master that part of your life. You get to choose. Not everybody wants the same things. Not everybody wants a bikini body, or a trip around the world, or the responsibility of running a business or… you name it. And that's OK. But you need to realise that it's a choice. You need to commit to your chosen outcome – over and above everything else you could choose – while consistently implementing the strategy that can help you get it done and investing the time, energy, effort, money and everything else required to achieve it.

Despite infertility and miscarriage, the outcome of having a baby, in this day and age, is also a consequence of one's various choices. When I first began clinical practice, the technology that could enable a couple (or individual) to have a baby was still somewhat inaccessible by most people. But these days, there are so many more options, as well as increased accessibility to these options. So much, in fact, that it can be overwhelming. But it all comes at a cost (physical, emotional and financial). Therefore, the first step on this journey is to be real with yourself – what do *you* want more: a baby or a way of having a baby? There's no one right answer to that. It's a personal decision. It's always a choice. And if you don't choose the things that will help support all your other choices in the process (even if you need IVF or donors or whatever else), you're choosing to remain stuck right where you are. Choice and personal responsibility – these two decisions change the game (in many cases, so completely that a previous situation can become unrecognisable). Whatever you do, be clear about one thing: excuses don't deliver babies.

Knowing something and not implementing it is the same as not knowing it at all. This is so important it bears repeating: *If you know it, but you don't apply that knowledge, it's the same as not knowing it at all.* Without proper application, priceless information becomes useless information.

Half-heartedly 'trying' or coming up with creative excuses as to why the knowledge is so hard to implement won't get you your baby. You need to act on what you learn and what you know. Applying what you know is what delivers the real results we all seek. Action puts you firmly in your area of influence.

And in taking action, you must be consistent. You won't get fit by doing 1,000 push-ups once. We're talking regular, every-single-day action. We're talking doing your very best (not your 'full of excuses' best) to persistently live the actions I prescribe – even if it means pushing yourself out of your comfort zone. Your comfort zone also doesn't deliver babies. Creating a healthy baby requires full commitment to your health and fertility – as does raising one. So, consider this effort, focus, expense and whatever else you are about to go through now, your preparation to embrace your desired outcome and making your dreams come true. Ultimately though, all this is about so much more than your fertility or a baby. This is about you becoming everything you're destined be.

As the ancient Chinese proverb says, a journey of 1,000 miles begins with one single step. Right now, you're facing in the right direction, all you need to do is walk. This section is all about helping you begin taking those steps in order to arrive at your desired destination.

I'll be your highly skilled guide on these first few steps, pointing out the way. But it's your choice to decide to continue walking once you've finished this book. No one, not even your partner, the very person who's committed to creating your desired outcome with you, can do that for you. You must decide to take on my challenge and to take charge of yourself in the process. Conquering yourself along the way – that's what this is all about.

• EPIGENETICS AND THE HEROIN ADDICT SYNDROME •

I once had a woman in my clinic who was in complete despair, sobbing about the challenges she faced in trying to conceive. At one point she stopped and angrily blurted out: 'Well, maybe if I just start shooting up heroin then I'll have a baby!' I was in shock for a moment, thinking her comment was odd and random. She noticed the perplexed look on my face and explained: 'I mean, here I am. I lead a healthy lifestyle, I have a good diet, I take my supplements and I can't get pregnant, no matter how hard I try. Yet junkies are having perfectly healthy babies every day.' I'm happy to report I was able to help this woman and her husband conceive naturally, and they now have a gorgeous and healthy baby girl, but her comment really got me thinking. In different ways, I get this question every day. 'Why must I do any of this **!\$%**! when my sister, brother, mother, aunty, neighbour, friend, parrot, etc are doing all the wrong things and getting pregnant and having healthy babies?'

This is a great question. I've come to refer to this conundrum as the 'heroin addict syndrome'.

There are many ways of looking at it. Let's start with the fact that just because society deems a normal-looking baby to be perfectly healthy at birth doesn't mean this baby is truly healthy.

But more importantly, the short answer to why some people have trouble conceiving while others seem to do all the wrong things and still get pregnant lies in a field of science called epigenetics. This is a relatively new field and involves studying how our specific genes are affected by environmental factors and challenges. Our body's genetic response to its environmental triggers can and will in many cases change our body's ability to function as might be expected.

We've all heard about those people who chain smoke and never develop lung cancer. In contrast, there's that person who never smoked a cigarette in their life and dies of lung cancer at a relatively young age. This is epigenetics at work. While some people's weakness may be their lungs, or their immune system, for others reproductive function may be affected.

The good news is that these challenges are seldom permanent or immutable. Your daily choices over a relatively small period of concerted effort can create the optimal changes you're looking for. The key is to stop comparing yourself with other people. Their journey is not your journey.

What can you lose by taking charge of your fertility to create your own breakthrough? The worst-case scenario is that you, your partner and your prospective child will be healthier and better off for it. And there's more. A baby's health blueprint is set for life by eight weeks' gestation. At this point, a baby already has all their little organs and all their fingerprints. Their health potential and predispositions are in place for the rest of their lives. It's therefore safe to say a child's health becomes the lowest common denominator of both partners' health at the time of conception.[2,3] This is why the time to optimise your child's health is during the preconception preparation period and not during pregnancy – contrary to popular belief.

The truth is, if you want to dramatically increase your chances of taking home a healthy baby – despite infertility and miscarriage – you must give the egg and sperm the minimum amount of time they need to mature and form.[4,5,6,7] The egg's full maturation process, from primordial follicles (which are the eggs we're born with) to ovulatory follicles, occurs in two stages of approximately 120 days each. In other words, approximately eight months.[8,9] And despite sperm having an approximate development cycle of over 100 days, in some cases in clinical practice, I've seen a complete change in a man's sperm parameters take as many as three sperm cycles to fully occur.

The great news is that for a large percentage of couples, a few months can truly make all the difference – despite years and sometimes decades of infertility and miscarriage. This is the case for many of our patients, who have healthy babies even after almost all hope has been lost.

Our patients and their gorgeous babies are living proof that you have even more reason to focus on optimising your health and fertility over a period of at least 120 days prior to a conception attempt. It's this very step that will improve the health of the DNA (think epigenetics) being passed on to your child.[10,11] It will also decrease your risk of future complications and of course increase your chances of being able to conceive and take a healthy pregnancy to term.[12,13,14]

Your 120 days of preconception preparation and beyond, utilising my seven-step F.E.R.T.I.L.E. Method®, isn't 'wasting time' or 'waiting'. It's an incredibly proactive time where you will be implementing the 11 Pillars of Fertility Foundations™. Whether you're implementing an effective or ineffective strategy, the time will pass – and I know what will count towards the results you want. To those looking in from the outside, it may seem like the slow approach. It isn't. It is the inside-out, transformational approach. The path less travelled but the one with the compass that will stop you from going around in circles with no baby to show for all your efforts.

If you want this, working as a team through the challenges I've set for you is going to give you the best possible chance of realising your dream – in the fastest possible time frame.

By the end of this section, you'll know what you need to do and why you need to do it. One thing is for sure: you won't be able to hide behind not knowing. So, waste not another second; surrender and commit, fully and decisively, as if your life depended on it – because your prospective child's most likely does.

And again, if you get stuck or if, like me, you prefer personalised guidance on any major endeavour, you can always reach out to my team, or participate in a Natural Fertility Breakthrough Program™ information session to learn more about how we may be able to assist you. Register to attend a complimentary session here: http://thefertile.me/NFBPInfoSession.

The 11 Pillars of Fertility Foundations™

Our patients' success stories are testimony to our proven track record as is our 78.15% success rate. Through treatment programs based on the 11 Pillars of Fertility Foundations™ (the basis of the F.E.R.T.I.L.E. Method®), we've helped thousands of couples. And many of them conceived and delivered healthy babies after they'd been told by other specialists that they'd likely never do so.

The integrative and holistic fertility treatment we deliver uses a blend of therapies. It combines the best of Eastern and Western expertise to help you heal and strengthen your body and reproductive system. My team and I believe the methodical implementation of the 11 Pillars of Fertility Foundations™ is one of the main reasons we're able to repeatedly help couples (and individuals) overcome infertility and miscarriage.

These pillars represent the important factors (personal environment, lifestyle, general health, etc) which can directly and indirectly affect human reproduction. For some, our programs may require dramatic lifestyle changes in addition to thorough biochemical investigations that previously may have been neglected. But our approach provides a new way to view your and your partner's body, offering a proven, step-by-step methodology and effective strategy to support you in restoring your system closer to balance and health, thus naturally maximising fertility for a healthy conception.

Like a gardener who must exert great effort (removing weeds) and also exercise great patience (waiting for the flowers to bloom), you must work hard to let go of everything that no longer serves you (your weeds) and be patient (while always proactively working towards your outcome). You must courageously open yourself up to a new level of awareness and willingness regarding your physical, mental, emotional and even spiritual nourishment. Sometimes, we must break down before we can break through.

This is so much more than a fertility program. It's not just for couples who wish to overcome infertility and miscarriage. Our process is an essential toolkit for anyone wishing to become the best version of themselves while preparing for a healthy conception and baby.

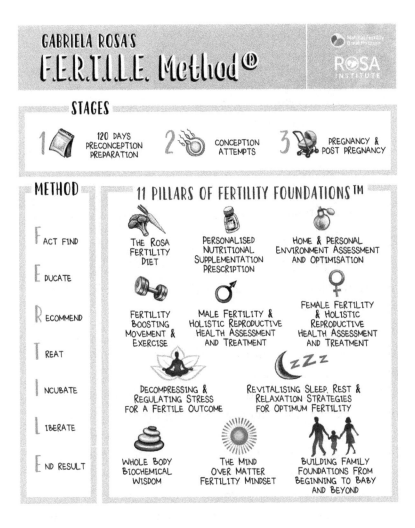

The 11 Pillars of Fertility Foundations™ encompass:

1. The Rosa Fertility Diet

2. Personalised Nutritional Supplementation Prescription

3. Home and Personal Environment Assessment and Optimisation

4. Fertility-boosting Movement and Exercise

5. Male Fertility and Holistic Reproductive Health Assessment and Treatment

6. Female Fertility and Holistic Reproductive Health Assessment and Treatment

7. Decompressing and Regulating Stress for a Fertile Outcome

8. Revitalising Sleep, Rest and Relaxation Strategies for Optimum Fertility

9. Whole Body Biochemical Wisdom

10. The Mind Over Matter Fertility Mindset

11. Building Family Foundations from Beginning to Baby and Beyond

You may think that if you just do some of the work, such as improve your diet or lifestyle, and take some supplements, that will be enough, but it isn't. The foundation of a building is its most important part. It's critical to build your fertility foundations. You must make sure these foundations – all of them – are as strong as necessary. However, it's also important to acknowledge that foundations alone don't erect buildings. It's the 'halfway' approach, instead of a holistic and integrated solution to a complex issue, that keeps most couples going around in circles. When you go only halfway, or build only half of your foundations, you'll invariably be disappointed with your results in the long term. This is what most people do, and then, feeling hopeless, they abandon the very foundations they've spent precious time, effort, energy and money building. They end up trying something new, mistakenly thinking that the huge amount of effort didn't result in anything, rather than applying a laser focus and a winning (though seemingly slow) strategy to achieve their objectives.

In any building endeavour, you must be fully committed to the entire process, otherwise you'll have an incomplete project to show for your efforts. You need an 'all in' approach to avoid lacklustre results. Ignore well-meaning friends and family who think you're crazy and going overboard with 'everything' that you're doing. If the bare minimum effort would work in your specific situation, you wouldn't be reading this book in the first place. If they 'decrease your suffering' by letting you off the hook, you'll only endure more heartbreak in the long run – so we might as well roll up our sleeves and get to work. The time is now.

Let's begin.

References

1   We are working with Harvard University and The University of Sydney Biostatistics Faculty to complete the retrospective analysis of The Natural Fertility Breakthrough Program™ patient data. Our patients are mostly over 40 and have been trying unsuccessfully to conceive or take a healthy pregnancy to term for over two years. For the patients who complete The Natural Fertility Breakthrough Program™, our overall success rate is 78.15%. This is an extraordinary result given that couples who undergo IVF/ICSI treatment typically see a 25–30% success rate. The full analysis and our official report will be published in early 2020.

2   Moore, K., et al., *The Developing Human: Clinically Oriented Embryology*. 9th ed. 2013, Philadelphia: Saunders.

3   Tortora, G.J., et al., *Principles of Anatomy and Physiology*. 14th ed. 2014, United States of America: Wiley.

4   Chavarro, J.E., et al., Diet and lifestyle in the prevention of ovulatory disorder infertility. *Obstetrics and Gynecology*, 2007. 110(5).

5   Chiu, Y.-H., et al., Diet and female fertility: Doctor, what should I eat? *Fertility and Sterility*, 2018. 110(4).

6   Mínguez-Alarcón, L., et al., Secular trends in semen parameters among men attending a fertility center between 2000 and 2017: Identifying potential predictors. *Environment International*, 2018. 121(Pt 2).

7   Nassan, F.L., et al., Diet and men's fertility: Does diet affect sperm quality? *Fertility and Sterility*, 2018. 110(4).

8   McGee, E.A., et al., Initial and cyclic recruitment of ovarian follicles. *Endocrine Reviews*, 2000. 21(2).

9   Wu, H., et al., Preconception urinary phthalate concentrations and sperm DNA methylation profiles among men undergoing IVF treatment: A cross-sectional study. *Human Reproduction* (Oxford, England), 2017. 32(11).

10   Barua, S., et al., Lifestyle, pregnancy and epigenetic effects. *Epigenomics*, 2015. 7(1).

11   Curley, J.P., et al., Epigenetics and the origins of paternal effects. *Hormones and Behavior*, 2011. 59(3).

12   Dean, S.V., et al., Importance of intervening in the preconception period to impact pregnancy outcomes. Nestle Nutrition Institute Workshop Series, 2013. 74.

13   Lassi, Z.S., et al., Preconception care: Screening and management of chronic disease and promoting psychological health. *Reproductive Health*, 2014. 11 (Suppl 3).

14   Tanvig, M., Offspring body size and metabolic profile – effects of lifestyle intervention in obese pregnant women. *Danish Medical Journal*, 2014. 61(7).

Prescription 1: Discover How Your Personal Environment Is Keeping You Infertile

'It is never a question of "if" someone is burdened with toxicants. It is a question of is their toxicant burden a causative factor in their illness, or an obstacle to cure.'

Walter Crinnion

According to the World Health Organization and the United Nations Environment Programme's *State of the Science of Endocrine Disrupting Chemicals*, 'close to 800 environmental chemicals are known or suspected to be capable of interfering with hormone receptors, hormone synthesis, or hormone conversion'. However, the toxic number of permutations when chemicals are combined is infinitely higher. These chemicals (and their toxic combinations) affect many systems in the body and can lead to infertility, birth defects, obesity, learning and memory difficulties, adult onset diabetes or cardiovascular disease, as well as a variety of other diseases.[1] And if this knowledge wasn't staggering enough, this report proceeds to state that only a fraction of these chemicals have been investigated in tests capable of identifying their effects on the endocrine system. I'm sure that the number of environmental chemicals in our environment grows daily, as well as their unknown compounded effects. This is a very real yet often hidden or ignored threat to the health and fertility status of the entire world's population. Lack of serious education and policy around this issue means it's a danger found in the heart of every home and workplace around the globe.

It's important to focus on the quality of indoor environments, as people spend more than 90% of their time indoors – and the things we bring into our living, work and recreational spaces contribute to disease.[2,3] Scientific research on toxic chemicals makes clear recommendations regarding the need to consider consumer products and building materials, including furniture, electronics, personal-care items, cleaning and pest-control products and floor and wall coverings – all of which are predominantly made from or heavily embedded with dangerous and toxic chemicals which are disguised as *safe*.[4,5] Now a Harvard T.H. Chan School of Public Health initiative Healthy Buildings For Health and their (May 2019) comprehensive report Homes for Health provides a wonderful summary of important considerations for health promoting indoor environments and further validates all the principles I share in this book.[6,7] Chemicals in any environment can leach, migrate, abrade, or off-gas from the various products in which they're found, and then it's only a matter of time until these chemicals cause disease, as well as infertility and miscarriage as toxins are inhaled, ingested or absorbed through the skin.[4,8] The bio-accumulative effect of most commercially available chemicals poses a serious risk to human health (general and reproductive) around the globe – and it's only due to a serious lack of public education, awareness and policy that this situation continues to be exacerbated each year, with new products entering the market for consumption.[9,10]

The Environmental Working Group revealed in one study[11] that there are thirty-eight secret chemicals in seventeen name-brand fragrance products. Some of these chemicals are known endocrine-disrupting chemicals (EDCs). That bottle of perfume you received for your birthday, or your partner's aftershave, is likely reducing your chances of taking home a healthy baby.[12,13,14] We must learn to protect ourselves and our families from these toxicants. Our fertility, health and long-term quality of life are categorically at stake.[15,16]

Persistent exposure to EDCs impacts your fertility on multiple levels. Contact with them can occur through touching them directly, drinking unfiltered water, ingesting tainted and processed food and even just breathing polluted air. It's impossible to completely avoid this type of chemical exposure. But you can minimise contact by knowing where many of the dangers can be found and making different choices.

In the following pages, you'll discover key fertility poisons you must familiarise yourself with and avoid if you want to transform your reproductive outcomes. But first, I'd like for you to understand the ways in which your personal environment might be keeping you infertile.

Some of the biggest fertility dangers in your personal environment will come in the form of seemingly inoffensive products.[17,18,19,20] And they can decrease your chances of taking home a healthy baby even if you're not directly in contact with them. For example, perhaps you have a cleaner, or your partner tinkers with chemicals somewhere. Think of hobbies and pastimes as well as occupational hazards that could be a factor here. Merely having chemicals in your immediate environment, such as that chock-a-block full laundry cupboard, is enough to pollute the air you breathe and negatively impact your and your partner's fertility.[19,21]

Chemicals found in plasticisers (plastics, non-stick surfaces, fabric protectors, etc), pesticides, fungicides, herbicides and industrial products all negatively impact endocrine function and therefore hormonal balance.[22,23] It's the job of the endocrine glands, such as the thyroid, ovaries and testicles, to control reproductive function. When this balance is upset because of improper biochemical communication, all sorts of problems can occur, including infertility and miscarriage.[24,25]

• HORMONES, ENDOCRINE DISRUPTORS AND BIOCHEMICAL MISCOMMUNICATION •

Hormones are signalling molecules that help the body function effectively. These biological substances are typically produced in one part of the body but have an effect on some other, distant area or system within the organism. This important biological task for which hormones are responsible occurs through a type of 'lock and key' mechanism that ensures metabolic processes operate in optimal balance. In simple terms, a specific hormone is meant for a distinctive cellular receptor site. Said hormones, being present or not, trigger a whole cascade of events through positive and/ or negative biofeedback loops that result in specific effects (positive, neutral or negative) within the biological organism, which is ultimately striving for homeostasis.[26,27]

The big reason for concern regarding EDCs is that they appear to the cell receptors, for which hormones are destined, as hormone 'lookalikes'. These endocrine impostors will lock onto a receptor site, and because they're not the hormones intended for that cell, they'll block a correct message or deliver an incorrect one, signalling the cell and directing it to do things in a way which may negatively impact optimal function, thus contributing to infertility and/or miscarriage.[28,29]

These chemicals can also alter normal hormone levels, stop or start key hormone production, and change the way in which hormones travel through the body or how they affect physiological functions such as those related to reproduction. They may even turn important activities on and off at the wrong times, or alter the level of gravity of critical messages. Most man-made chemicals found in our environment (including many discussed in this section) fall into the 'endocrine disruptor' category. Consequently, they may have a direct negative impact on your health and fertility if you don't take action to safeguard your and your partner's health.[28,30]

As mentioned, it's impossible to completely avoid endocrine disruptors, but there's a lot you can do to dramatically decrease your exposure to them in your home, and perhaps even in your work environment. Get them out of your personal environment. This is your most important task for today. This shouldn't take too long but it will make a world of positive difference to your health and fertility and the health of your prospective family. Avoid physical contact with and breathing in outgassed fumes from the chemical products stored in your cupboards. Look for those long, unpronounceable names or acronyms lurking in your sacred biospheres.[30,31]

Unfiltered water is also a big source of hazardous and unwanted chemicals in your environment.[32,33,34] Boiling your water will kill most (not all) harmful microorganisms. But it will also concentrate the chemicals it contains, so it's vital to invest in a good-quality water filter that attaches to your kitchen sink pipes or water spout with at most one micron filtration thickness (it can be placed either underneath or on top of the bench).[35,36,37] Jug filters are inadequate as they typically don't provide the fine filtration ideal to protect you and are made from plastic (which is full of potent endocrine disruptors).[38] Ceramic filters also aren't ideal because they're likely to develop internal mould, which is toxic and difficult to identify.[39,40]

Another way to reduce your direct exposure to toxic chemicals is to become a minimalist (at least in this area of your life). Buying and taking home fewer products of all types and choosing food with less packaging wherever possible is a great start. Also, not wearing shoes in the house will limit the number of toxic chemicals, bacteria and viruses you unwittingly bring into your home. Think about it. Your shoes step into public toilets, and walk on microparticles of animal faeces, and on chemicals found in certain types of flooring and the products used to clean them, and on the general dirt of public places. When you step into your own home wearing those same shoes, you bring all types of (endocrine-disrupting) chemicals and microorganisms into your home. This is something very simple to avoid.

So, if you don't bring cleaning products into your home, how will you keep your environment clean and germ free? Just like your grandma did more than fifty years ago, with old fashioned, simple and above all extremely safe and effective water, vinegar, eucalyptus or tea tree oil and bicarbonate of soda. Although there are many other options available in the market today, these are safe, relatively inexpensive, very effective and most importantly low toxicity options, which will help you remove some of the obstacles to your optimum fertility and thus improve your chances of taking home a healthy baby.

MIRACLE MOMENTS

• GIVE IT YOUR BEST SHOT •

KRISTINE AND BEN

For three years, my husband and I didn't use contraception. While we weren't exactly trying for a baby, we would have been happy if we got pregnant. Then we decided the time was right and we should actively try to get pregnant. After eighteen months of trying, with no result, we were starting to get worried, so we went to our local doctor.

She did the usual blood tests and suggested we see a fertility specialist. The specialist recommended exploratory surgery to find out what was happening. She said we had 'unexplained infertility'. We were incredibly disappointed. What could we do? What did that even mean?

Our local doctor was pushing for IVF because I was thirty-eight, and I kept being told over and over that time was running out. I was scared but I wasn't sure. We decided to do Gabriela's fertility assessment, and I couldn't believe how much more comprehensive it was compared to my previous two consultations, first with my local doctor and then with the fertility specialist. Gabriela's approaches really resonated with us, so we decided to join the Natural Fertility Breakthrough Program™.

We implemented everything Gabriela and her team recommended throughout each stage of the program. I was really hoping to conceive naturally; however, I was also open to the idea that if, after all the appropriate investigations, Gabriela deemed it necessary, we would go down the IVF path. It was definitely our last resort. So, we focused and we did... everything.

I was so surprised by how extensive Gabriela's testing protocol was – no one I'd seen before requested anything even close to what she asked in order to holistically treat our case. Finally, someone was checking everything. I felt a peace of mind regarding my fertility and the whole journey to baby that I hadn't experienced since the very first couple of months being with Ben. The volley of testing found many more minor factors that were reducing our fertility. Some important additions to the puzzle included subclinical hypothyroidism and a mutation in the MTHFR gene. These factors, in combination with so many others in our case, including sperm-parameter abnormalities, helped explain our inability to conceive. I finally became aware of how everything was interlinked and how it was all contributing to my hormone imbalances and the variable length of my cycles. I also became aware of the luteal phase defect that may have been impacting implantation for us and causing shortened cycles with poor egg maturation, as well as my ongoing problems with low B12 and energy levels.

So many aspects of both our health improved throughout the program. I was thrilled. It took us about six months to improve my cycle enough to start trying to conceive. Then I got pregnant naturally on our second attempt. We were amazed. We couldn't have achieved this without all the work we did and the help of Gabriela and her team.

For more information on what you need to avoid and what else you could use in your personal environment, see Tables 3.1 and 3.2.

Table 3.1: EDCs commonly found in products in and around the home[41,42,43,44,45,46,47]

Category	Unsafe – AVOID
Cleaning	Ammonia – Ammonium lauryl sulfate (ALS) Artificial/synthetic fragrances (parfum) Benzotriazole Chlorine (lye) Diethyl phthalate Dyes Formaldehyde Glycol ethers – 2-butoxyethanol Nanoparticles Phosphates Phthalates Propylene Sodium hydroxide Sodium laureth sulfate (SLES) Triclosan (antibacterial) Zeolites
Laundry	Alkylphenol ethoxylates Ammonia Artificial/synthetic fragrances (parfum) Bleach (sodium hypochlorite) Galaxolide Monoethanolamine (MEA) Petroleum distillates (napthas) Phosphates Phthalates Optical brighteners Quaternary ammonium compounds (quats) SLES Tonalide Triclosan (antibacterial)
Personal hygiene & personal care	Alumina Aluminium Antiperspirants Artificial/synthetic fragrances (parfum) Benzalkonium chloride BHA/BHT Cadmium

Personal hygiene & personal care *[continued]*	Camphor Carrageenan DPB FD&C colours Flavour Formaldehyde Glycerin (non-vegetable derived) Isopropyl Microbeads Mineral oil Musks Nanoparticles Octocrylene Parabens Paraffin PEG Petrolatum Phenoxyethanol Phthalates Propylene glycol Retinoic acid Retinyl palmitate Siloxanes SLES Sodium fluoride Sodium lauryl sulfate Sodium saccharin Talc TEA/DEA Toluene Triclosan (antibacterial)
Pest control	Commercially available pesticides and herbicides, especially those containing glyphosate or DEET
Food storage & kitchen utensils	All plastics, including BPA and BPA-free plastics, Aluminium Ceramic-coated cookware Non-stick coatings (even if PFOA & PTFE free) PFOA PTFE Teflon

Table 3.2: Suggested alternatives to reduce EDCs in your personal environment [48,49,50]

Category	Alternatives
Cleaning	Bicarbonate of soda (baking soda) Castile soap Citrus peels Coconut- and sugar-based nonionic surfactants Essential oils* Salt Sodium carbonate Sodium silicate Vinegar Water
Laundry	Bicarbonate of soda (baking soda) Castile soap Coconut- and sugar-based nonionic surfactants Essential oils* Soda ash Sodium percarbonate Vinegar Water
Personal hygiene & personal care	Alkylpolyglucosides (APGs) Apple cider vinegar Beeswax Bicarbonate of soda (baking soda) Castile soap Coconut oil Cold-pressed oils (almond, olive) Essential oils* Glycerin (vegetable derived) Glycine extracts Glycolic acid Grain alcohol Shea butter Soda ash Sodium coco sulfate Xanthan gum White vinegar

Pest control	Bicarbonate of soda (baking soda) Castile soap Diatomaceous earth Essential oils* Honey Sugar
Food storage & kitchen utensils	Cast-iron/enamel-coated cookware Glass storage/baking containers Stainless-steel storage containers/pots/pans/cooking utensils Wooden chopping boards/utensils (be mindful of glues used)

* It's vital to be aware that some essential oils are contraindicated in pregnancy and therefore best avoided when trying to conceive (see Table 3.3, which is by no means an exhaustive list). Always consult a qualified aromatherapist if in doubt about the use of any essential oil in your specific situation. However, direct contact with essential oils should be avoided, as many of the concentrated oils of these plants have abortifacient and other properties incompatible with conception and pregnancy.

Table 3.3 – Essential oils contraindicated in pregnancy and when trying to conceive

Essential oils to avoid[51]		
Aniseed	Cumin	Rue
Aniseed myrtle	Cypress	Sage
Atlas cedarwood	Fennel	Savin
Basil	Hyssop	Spanish lavender
Birch	Indian dill seed	Star anise
Blue cypress	Jasmine	Sweet birch
Buchu ct. diosphenol	Juniper berry	Sweet marjoram
Buchu ct. pulegone	Mugwort	Tansy
Camphor	Myrrh	Tarragon
Carrot seed	Neem	Thuja
Cassia	Oregano	Thyme
Cinnamon	Parsley seed or leaf	Western red cedar
Clary sage	Pennyroyal	Wintergreen
Clove	Peppermint	Winter savoury
Costus	Rosemary	Wormwood

• HOW TO CLEAN YOUR HOME WITH JUST THREE (SAFE) INGREDIENTS •

You need only three ingredients to clean your home (other than water, of course): vinegar, bicarbonate of soda and, for the extreme germaphobes out there, tea tree or eucalyptus oil (I've used tea tree oil, preferably bought in glass, for years in my laundry, kitchen and bathrooms, with great delight).

The simplest recipe is two parts water to one part vinegar. Mix it in a spray bottle (glass is ideal) and use it for cleaning work surfaces, toilets, bathtubs and more. Before using, be sure to spot-check to avoid damage to surfaces. For stubborn stains, use a little (or a lot of) bicarbonate of soda paste with a little vinegar or water.

Microfibre cloths (without silver particles or nanotechnology) can also be extremely helpful. I don't recommend nanotechnology-embedded cleaning cloths, as anything with nanoparticles or heavy metals could potentially play a role in endocrine disruption (I discuss heavy metals and other toxins, as well as how to protect your health and fertility from them, in more detail in our Environmental Toxins infographics: http://thefertile.me/infographics).

I've also assembled a special interactive portal for this book, which you can access at http://thefertile.me/BreakthroughBook. In it you'll find many extra resources, including some of the cleaning and pest-control recipes previously published in some of my other books (available at http://thefertile.me/books).

MIRACLE MOMENTS

• ACT PREGNANT NOW •
STEPHANIE AND DARREN

Before joining Gabriela's Natural Fertility Breakthrough Program, we thought our diet and lifestyle were healthy, and we were taking supplements. However, we'd been trying to conceive for three years, and we were becoming despondent. We truly thought it was never going to happen for us. We are holistically minded and went along to a local naturopath. She didn't do any testing; she made some suggestions and gave us some drops to take. We kept visiting her for a few months, but without success.

Then we did one of Gabriela's Fertility Challenges™ and were impressed with the quality of the information she provided. So, we decided to join the Natural Fertility Breakthrough Program™, and our lives changed dramatically. At this point, regardless of the worst-case scenario of not being able to conceive, we were healthier, happier, content, calm, peaceful and connected as a couple. We felt so much better and had higher energy levels. It was life-changing. We also understood clearly why we couldn't conceive and why, in the years we had been trying, no one else had got to the bottom of our issue until we started our treatment with Gabriela's team.

We started taking charge of the things we could influence – our home environment, our lifestyle and our health. We started eating better food and a wider variety, but more importantly we started eating the right types of food. We finally understood what healthy really meant.

I stopped drinking bottled water. My cycle improved dramatically. I had less pain, my cycles were more regular, and shorter, and my flow wasn't so heavy anymore. Our energy levels were huge. We were bouncing out of our skin and we didn't even need coffee.

We had some more tests and diagnostics done, and I came back with a positive chlamydia result. I'd obviously been positive for a long time, and it had caused scarring in my tubes. Gabriela insisted that I go to my doctor to get my tubes tested, despite no doctor having ever suggested it in my three years of infertility, and I was met with resistance when I asked. If it wasn't for Gabriela being absolutely adamant it had to be done, I probably would have just accepted my doctor's lack of interest in checking it further. The testing showed both my tubes to be completely blocked. Without that test, I would probably still be childless today because, as Gabriela says, we would have run out of time altogether. Now, with the clarity we were missing all along, we understood this meant our only option was IVF.

At last, for the first time in three years, we felt empowered with the knowledge we gained. It helped us to stop panicking and worrying. We completely trusted Gabriela and did everything she advised to prepare for a successful cycle. We weren't in the dark regarding our fertility anymore. There was no little voice in the back of my head saying, 'What if it never happens?' because I just knew that when everything was right and our bodies were ready, we could confidently take the next step towards conception. We did all the things that Gabriela asked us to do in our preconception preparation ahead of our IVF cycle. We knew we had to get all our minor factors right and not just bypass my blocked tubes before starting on the emotional and expensive IVF journey.

It all boiled down to Gabriela's brilliant advice to my husband and me 'to act pregnant now to get pregnant later'. Now it all makes perfect sense. This helped our bodies and minds get prepared for pregnancy. By following Gabriela and her team's expert guidance, in our very first IVF cycle we created three perfect embryos. The first one transferred had me give birth to my beautiful baby girl, Arianna. A couple of years later, sweet little Georgia was born, and we still have one miracle baby in the freezer. We are so grateful for the day we found you, Gabriela. Thank you for everything.

Fertility Reset Prescription 1: Throw out the chemicals

For the sake of your optimum fertility, get a giant garbage bag and place into it every bottle of commercially available cleaning and pest-control product in your house. As a second (potentially more difficult yet very important) step, be sure to tackle your make-up and personal-care-regime items when you are feeling brave too.

The big issue with all these chemicals is that even if you don't personally use them, if they're used in your environment, the residue (or volatile component, especially in the case of fragrances contained within most products) will still negatively affect your and your partner's fertility. For example, research shows that sperm is strongly affected by fragrances in perfumes, colognes, aftershave preparations and more.[52,53,54] The chemical dangers in one's environment are far more insidious and problematic than meets the eye when it comes to a couple's fertility.

Most local councils consider a garbage bag full of cleaning and chemical products hazardous material as far as disposal is concerned. So, you may need to contact your local authorities to find out the best way to dispose of these. They shouldn't be going into the ordinary landfill, as they're highly toxic and can also negatively impact the environment. Another alternative is to donate such products to homeless or women's shelters or other organisations that might use them.

Some people may argue this is an extreme approach. But if all the evidence regarding chemicals' endocrine disruptive abilities can be easily found in the scientific literature and reports from some of the most prestigious institutions and organisations around the world and that isn't enough to convince those people, then I don't know what is. Others claim that making the required changes to optimise fertility is too hard, but my patients assure me every day that long-standing infertility and recurrent miscarriage is infinitely harder. My patients also prove that not only is it possible to implement this approach, it's also an essential part of a comprehensive and winning strategy to achieve thriving health and transform reproductive challenges, even when other treatments have failed.

Resources

For more information on safe products and other valuable resources to help you finally take home a healthy baby, visit the Fertility Breakthrough interactive book portal at http://thefertile.me/BreakthroughBook.

References

1   WHO, et al., State of the science of endocrine disrupting chemicals – 2012. 2013.

2   Mitro, S.D., et al., Consumer product chemicals in indoor dust: A quantitative meta-analysis of U.S. studies. *Environmental Science & Technology*, 2016. 50(19).

3   Zota, A.R., et al., Reducing chemical exposures at home: Opportunities for action. *Journal of Epidemiology and Community Health*, 2017. 71(9).

4   Wang, A., et al., Environmental influences on reproductive health, the importance of chemical exposures. *Fertility and Sterility*, 2016. 106(4).

5   Zheng, X., et al., Flame retardants on the surface of phones and personal computers. *The Science of the Total Environment*, 2017. 609.

6   Harvard T. H. Chan School for Public Health, Homes for Health, May 2019. https://homes.forhealth.org

7   Hipwell, A.E., et al., Exposure to non-persistent chemicals in consumer products and fecundability: A systematic review. *Human Reproduction Update*, 2019. 25(1).

8   Silins, I., et al., Combined toxic exposures and human health: biomarkers of exposure and effect. *International Journal of Environmental Research and Public Health*, 2011. 8(3).

9   Budnik, L.T., et al., Diagnosis, monitoring and prevention of exposure-related non-communicable diseases in the living and working environment: DiMoPEx-project is designed to determine the impacts of environmental exposure on human health. *Journal of Occupational Medicine and Toxicology* (London, England), 2018. 13.

10   Genuis, S.J., et al., Toxicant exposure and bioaccumulation: A common and potentially reversible cause of cognitive dysfunction and dementia. *Behavioural Neurology*, 2015. 2015.

11   Sarantis, H., et al., Not so sexy: The health risks of secret chemicals in fragrance. 2010.

12   Chow, E., et al., Cosmetics use and age at menopause: Is there a connection? *Fertility and Sterility*, 2016. 106(4).

13   Martina, C.A., et al., Lifestyle behaviors associated with exposures to endocrine disruptors. *Neurotoxicology*, 2012. 33(6).

14   Zota, A.R., et al., The environmental injustice of beauty: Framing chemical exposures from beauty products as a health disparities concern. *American Journal of Obstetrics and Gynecology*, 2017. 217(4).

15   Bijlsma, N., et al., *Environmental chemical assessment in clinical practice: Unveiling the elephant in the room. International Journal of Environmental Research and Public Health*, 2016. 13(2).

16   Hernández, A.F., et al., Human exposure to chemical mixtures: Challenges for the integration of toxicology with epidemiology data in risk assessment. *Food and Chemical Toxicology*: An International Journal Published for the British Industrial Biological Research Association, 2017. 103.

17   Bonde, J.P., et al., The epidemiologic evidence linking prenatal and postnatal exposure to endocrine disrupting chemicals with male reproductive disorders: A systematic review and meta-analysis. *Human Reproduction Update*, 2017. 23(1).

18   Craig, Z.R., et al., Pretty good or pretty bad? The ovary and chemicals in personal care products. *Toxicological Sciences*: *An Official Journal of the Society of Toxicology*, 2018. 162(2).

19   Dionisio, K.L., et al., Exploring consumer exposure pathways and patterns of use for chemicals in the environment. *Toxicology Reports*, 2015. 2.

20   Kim, D., et al., Reproductive disorders among cosmetologists and hairdressers: A meta-analysis. *International Archives of Occupational and Environmental Health*, 2016. 89(5).

21   Lucattini, L., et al., A review of semi-volatile organic compounds (SVOCs) in the indoor environment: Occurrence in consumer products, indoor air and dust. *Chemosphere*, 2018. 201.

22   De Coster, S., et al., Endocrine-disrupting chemicals: Associated disorders and mechanisms of action. *Journal of Environmental and Public Health*, 2012.

23   Street, M.E., et al., Current knowledge on endocrine disrupting chemicals (EDCs) from animal biology to humans, from pregnancy to adulthood: Highlights from a national Italian meeting. *International Journal of Molecular Sciences*, 2018. 19(6).

24   Gore, A.C., et al., EDC-2: The Endocrine Society's second scientific statement on endocrine-disrupting chemicals. *Endocrine Reviews*, 2015. 36(6).

25   Swaen, G.M.H., et al., Impact of changes in human reproduction on the incidence of endocrine-related diseases. *Critical Reviews in Toxicology*, 2018.

26   Tata, J.R., One hundred years of hormones. *EMBO Reports*, 2005. 6(6).

27   Tsigos, C., et al., Stress, endocrine physiology and pathophysiology, in *Endotext*, K.R. Feingold, et al., Editors. 2000, MDText.com, Inc.: South Dartmouth (MA).

28   Sifakis, S., et al., Human exposure to endocrine disrupting chemicals: Effects on the male and female reproductive systems. *Environmental Toxicology and Pharmacology*, 2017. 51.

29   Stel, J., et al., The role of epigenetics in the latent effects of early life exposure to obesogenic endocrine disrupting chemicals. *Endocrinology*, 2015. 156(10).

30   Menezo, Y., Jr., et al., The negative impact of the environment on methylation/epigenetic marking in gametes and embryos: A plea for action to protect the fertility of future generations. *Molecular Reproduction and Development*, 2019.

31   Annamalai, J., et al., Endocrine disrupting chemicals in the atmosphere: Their effects on humans and wildlife. *Environment International*, 2015. 76.

32   Di Nisio, A., et al., Water and soil pollution as determinant of water and food quality/contamination and its impact on male fertility. *Reproductive Biology and Endocrinology: RB&E*, 2019. 17(1).

33   Leusch, F.D.L., et al., Transformation of endocrine disrupting chemicals, pharmaceutical and personal care products during drinking water disinfection. *The Science of the Total Environment*, 2019. 657.

34   Wee, S.Y., et al., Endocrine disrupting compounds in drinking water
      supply system and human health risk implication. *Environment
      International*, 2017. 106.

35   Egorov, A.I., et al., Exposures to drinking water chlorination by-products in a
      Russian city. *International Journal of Hygiene and Environmental Health*, 2003.
      206(6).

36   King, W.D., et al., Exposure assessment in epidemiologic studies of
      adverse pregnancy outcomes and disinfection byproducts. *Journal of
      Exposure Analysis and Environmental Epidemiology*, 2004. 14(6).

37   Matsui, T., et al., Removal effect of the water purifier for home use against
      Cryptosporidium parvum oocysts. *The Journal of Veterinary Medical Science*,
      2004. 66(8).

38   Honeycutt, J.A., et al., Effects of water bottle materials and filtration on
      Bisphenol A content in laboratory animal drinking water. *Journal of the
      American Association for Laboratory Animal Science: JAALAS*, 2017. 56(3).

39   Mellor, J., et al., Modeling the sustainability of a ceramic water filter
      intervention. *Water Research*, 2014. 49.

40   Wingender, J., et al., Biofilms in drinking water and their role as reservoir
      for pathogens. *International Journal of Hygiene and Environmental Health*,
      2011. 214(6).

41   Fourth National Report on Human Exposure to Environmental
      Chemicals Update. 2018.

42   Bennike, N.H., et al., Fragrance contact allergens in 5588 cosmetic
      products identified through a novel smartphone application. *Journal of the
      European Academy of Dermatology and Venereology: JEADV*, 2018. 32(1).

43   Chiang, C., et al., Environmental contaminants affecting fertility and
      somatic health. *Seminars in Reproductive Medicine*, 2017. 35(3).

44   Steinemann, A., National prevalence and effects of multiple chemical
      sensitivities. *Journal of Occupational and Environmental Medicine*, 2018. 60(3).

45   Vandenberg, L.N., et al., Hormones and endocrine-disrupting chemicals:
      Low-dose effects and nonmonotonic dose responses. *Endocrine Reviews*,
      2012. 33(3).

46   WHO, et al., State of the science of endocrine disrupting chemicals –
      2012. 2013.

47   Chemicals in the Fourth Report: Updated Tables, March 2018.

48   Environmental Working Group, EWG's Guide to Healthy Cleaning.
      2019. www.ewg.org/guides/cleaners

49   Environmental Working Group, Skin Deep Cosmetics Database. 2019.
      www.ewg.org/skindeep

50   Zoeller, R.T., et al., Endocrine-disrupting chemicals and public
      health protection: a statement of principles from the Endocrine Society.
      Endocrinology, 2012. 153(9).

51   Battaglia, S., *The Complete Guide to Aromatherapy*. 3rd ed.
      Vol. 1 – Foundations & Materia Medica. 2018, QLD,
      Australia: Black Pepper Creative.

52   Bloom, M.S., et al., Associations between urinary phthalate
      concentrations and semen quality parameters in a general population.
      Human Reproduction (Oxford, England), 2015. 30(11).

53   Hauser, R., et al., Urinary phthalate metabolite concentrations and
      reproductive outcomes among women undergoing in vitro fertilization:
      Results from the EARTH Study. *Environmental Health Perspectives*, 2016.
      124(6).

54   Schettler, T., Human exposure to phthalates via consumer products.
      International Journal of Andrology, 2006. 29(1).

CHAPTER 9

Prescription 2: Take The Right Supplements

'I am my own work of art.'

Madonna

Supplementation is an important pillar in my 11 Pillars of Fertility Foundations™ and F.E.R.T.I.L.E. Method®. But whenever someone who hasn't done any of my programs asks me, 'I'm trying to have a baby – what supplements should I take?' I help them understand why self-prescription is a terrible idea. You and your partner are unique. And effective fertility treatment is complex and must consider many aspects of a person's health. The solution is never as simple as reading a prescription from a book or an online post.

Before we make even the first, most basic recommendations in terms of what nutrients our patients require, my team and I do an intense amount of work over many hours to understand clearly and in great detail where they have been, where they are now and where they need to go on their fertility journey in order to transform their results.

That first step entails a massive fact-finding mission. Before our team prescribes a seemingly inoffensive multivitamin (at any given time, we have five different ones in our dispensary, each for specific circumstances), a couple must first submit their fully completed comprehensive health and fertility appraisal questionnaire. They must also complete our F.E.R.T.I.L.E. Diagnostic Assessment™ online. Then I ask for all the results of previous investigations they have on hand from at least the last two years. Once we have all this information, we put together that couple's personalised treatment. Part of this step involves entering every examination a couple has ever undertaken in a comprehensive spreadsheet. This helps us make important clinical determinations regarding further diagnostics and treatment. And this is just the beginning. We're still a long way from the baby at this stage, but at least we're already facing in the right direction. Now we must walk.

Next, we put together a preliminary prescription for our first session with the couple – what we in-house affectionately named The Fertility Alignment™. During this session, we spend another hour or two further refining both partners' treatment. Once this is done, we deliver the prescription, along with our reasoning.

And the work continues. At each session during a couple's participation in our customised and personalised treatment program, we observe and further identify what changes, large or small, may be needed in their prescription. This isn't a static process of setting and forgetting; it evolves with the couple.

Other practitioners may immediately recommend treatment (including an IVF prescription) without doing the full fact-find that we heavily invest time and effort into as part of the F.E.R.T.I.L.E. Method® – but we know our method is the very best (and, in the long term, the fastest) way to help create the results we're well known for.

Again, I want a baby for my patients as much as they want one for themselves, and this is why I absolutely abhor self-prescription. It leaves too much to chance and can ultimately mean the difference between having a baby or not.

Self-prescription is akin to taking cold or flu medicine when what you really need is open-heart surgery. Don't undertake the important step of supplementation without the proper knowledge, supervision and expertise.

• TOP SEVEN REASONS WHY
YOU SHOULD NEVER SELF-PRESCRIBE •

1. Self-prescription invariably leads you to take the wrong supplements for your specific situation, so you end up wasting precious time and money.

2. Supplements you buy over the counter (in a supermarket, pharmacy, health food store or online) without a specific prescription often end up being 'sugar lollies' – either they have no effect or they have the wrong effect.[1,2,3]

3. The wrong supplementation and herbal medicines can further exacerbate imbalances in your biochemistry, negatively impacting hormonal balance and thus egg and sperm quality as well – leading to further wasted time.

4. For the most part, prospective parents won't have access to appropriate practitioner-only products because they require a practitioner's prescription. Also, we're constantly changing the brands we use when better formulations come into the market. It's vital to stay up to date with the latest developments in science (based on clinical trials conducted around the world) – and it's easy to fall into the trap of not knowing what you don't know in this arena.

5. Different situations can require drastically different approaches and clinically meaningful formulations with significantly disparate therapeutic doses. And you won't be able to figure these things out on your own.[4,5]

6. You won't be able to discern good- versus bad-quality products and/or ingredient-form variations within products. Some over-the-counter products use more excipients than active ingredients, and many are less-than-health-promoting adjuncts such as petroleum derivatives and other industrial chemicals, eg, acetone, ammonia and formaldehyde – all incredibly toxic EDCs.[6,7,8,9]

7. Typically, the cheaper the supplement, the less effective it is. A classic case of 'you get what you pay for'.

Just thinking about where to source your supplements leads to a Pandora's box of concerns. Good-quality products use biologically activated forms of vitamins and minerals. Cheaper products may substitute folinic acid or methylfolate for folic acid (toxic in high doses and low quality), or calcium amino acid chelate for calcium carbonate. Low-quality products are typically made from allergenic and sometimes even endocrine-disrupting excipients, including soy, corn, gluten and lactose, that should be avoided as much as possible. Cheap supplements may also suffer from lack of batch monitoring for safety and efficacy over time. Ultimately, the time wasted on the wrong strategy leads to one thing – a lack of a baby.

Couples from all over the world consult with us because they want the very best team to work on their case. And when dealing with a time-sensitive, life-altering circumstance, I did the same. When I received the news that my dad had been diagnosed with late-stage colorectal cancer which had metastasised to the liver and that he'd need twenty-eight sessions of oral chemotherapy, twenty-eight sessions of radiation, three-quarters of his liver removed and about forty centimetres of bowel resected before undergoing twelve rounds of intravenous chemotherapy, I didn't say to him: 'Here, Dad, let me give you a couple of supplements to take.'

I knew that he needed some serious nutritional guidance and emotional support. I also knew that there wasn't enough time for me to catch up on the latest cancer research (research others had spent twenty-plus years on). So, what did I do? I searched the globe and found the very best integrative medicine specialists, and I'm grateful I did. My dad worked with two amazing professionals approximately 16,000 kilometres away from where he lived. How did they manage to treat him from so far away? The same way we treat our patients – via online consultations.

We spent the next twelve months going through the journey outlined with the support of the two incredible specialists. The result? My dad's main oncologist couldn't believe his progress and response to treatment. It turns out that medical oncologists dealing with patients with cancer as advanced as my dad's seldom see these types of responses. My dad barely had any side effects that result from such heavy duty treatment. He was able to manage these and so much more because of the comprehensive, integrative and holistic approach that was personalised to him. Because my dad's overall response was so good, halfway through the treatment, his oncologist decided he was happy with only nine instead of twelve intravenous chemotherapy sessions and just asked to keep monitoring him.

My dad has always been disciplined, and he kept up an impeccable health regime with the support of the health team we assembled for him. Before his second lot of monitoring with a new doctor due to relocation (after those nine sessions, the investigations included a radioactive contrast PET scan, an MRI and blood tests), during his initial consultation, the oncologist wasn't exactly encouraging and seemed to be preparing him for the fact that he'd need to have further treatment. This would have meant that not all the cancer was eradicated and the whole thing would begin again. But I'm thrilled to say that when the reports came in, the doctor's words were: 'I'm happy just to keep monitoring you. Everything is clear. This is marvellous.' Such is the power of a great team, the right expertise and a willingness to 'do what it takes'.

Don't underestimate the importance of having the right team on your side – for my dad, it meant the difference between life and death, and for you, it could mean the difference between the status quo and a new life.

MIRACLE MOMENTS

• GET THE RIGHT NOURISHMENT •
KARLA AND DAVE

I was thirty-one years old and we'd been married for about a year when I miscarried at ten weeks. A local naturopath advised us that the issue was that Dave had poor sperm morphology. After a couple more miscarriages under the care of this naturopath, we decided it was time for a change. Fortunately, we fell pregnant a few months later, and I carried our daughter, Pearl, to full term.

It had taken a while to get our first child, and now I was almost thirty-five years old, so we started trying again. I got pregnant and we were excited that we'd be parents again. Sadly, at seventeen weeks I miscarried. It took us a long time to recover from this trauma, but we managed to pick ourselves up. We got healthy, and I fell pregnant again. Just one week later I miscarried. I couldn't believe it – I was devastated.

I knew that something was wrong. I had done lots of research and read about Gabriela. I knew that she looked at the physical, biochemical and emotional aspects of her patients, so I booked us in for a consultation.

I really liked that she took a scientific approach. It was the most rigorous, comprehensive, involved testing process that I could imagine. We found out that there was nothing majorly wrong with Dave (but there were many minor factors at work). However, I was severely malnourished and my amino acid levels were incredibly low.

I was a vegetarian and relied on carbohydrates for nourishment. I really didn't want to introduce meat into my diet, so Gabriela devised a tailored program of vitamins and minerals and a custom-prescribed amino-acid formulation based on the tests I'd done. She warned me that it could take a long time to get back to full health, but I trusted her advice and started on her program.

I accidentally got pregnant a short time later, and carried our baby, Autumn, to term. Autumn had a terminal brain condition and died when she was just two months old. This was the most difficult thing I had ever had to go through in my life.

By now, Dave had had enough and wasn't keen to continue trying. It was so difficult for us – the losses, the pain and despair. As a kid, I was a horse rider, and whenever I fell off, I remembered my mother urging me to 'get back on the horse', so I knew I couldn't stop. I still had the strength to try again.

The lifestyle and diet changes we learned on Gabriela's program had stuck. We were in good health; my nutrition was great. Five months after Autumn died, I got pregnant and went on to give birth to Gigi, a healthy, happy girl.

At thirty-nine years old, when Gigi was six months old, I accidentally got pregnant again. Now, our family is complete with a robust, healthy boy: Phoenix. Gabriela has been like a friend as well as a trusted advisor during this whole process. The program requires lifestyle changes, some very big, but the results for us have been truly life-changing.

Having said all this, I want to give you something you can begin implementing now: my favourite healing elixir – the whole lemon drink. It will support your body's biochemistry in many wonderful ways. My colleague Peter De Ruyter shared it with me many years ago, and I've prescribed it for my patients with great results for years. If you don't yet have the right supplement prescription, you can do something great for your body in the meantime. This food-based, therapeutic blend helps to improve immunological and overall health. It will also get you started on boosting liver health. This important organ is responsible for over 500 different activities in the body, including cleansing, creating hormonal balance, manufacturing new cellular building blocks and much more – all of which eventually translates into healthier eggs, sperm and baby.

• THE WHOLE LEMON DRINK RECIPE •

Preparation time: 5 minutes
Serves: 1 person (2.5 servings)

Ingredients:

1 whole organic, homegrown, pesticide- and wax-free lemon

1 ½ cups *filtered* water (all your water must be filtered by a good-quality water filter – this is critical for your optimum health and fertility)

2–3 tablespoons of raw coconut butter or MCT oil or liquid fish oil high in DHA (not cod liver oil)

1 tablespoon of sunflower lecithin

1 x 500 IU capsule of vitamin E (whole into the blender)

1 knob of fresh ginger (approximately golf-ball size)

Method:

Wash the lemon well and scrub it to remove any wax or residues.

Cut the lemon into small pieces and put it in the blender (skin on).

Add the rest of the ingredients to the blender. Blend for 2 to 3 minutes – to the texture you enjoy. The longer you blend, the smoother it becomes. Add extra water if you'd like it less thick.

How to take the whole lemon drink:

Consume half of the liquid before or with breakfast and half before or with dinner (the second half needs to be stored in a clean glass container in the fridge).

Always consume the total amount within twenty-four hours to prevent rancidity and too much oxidation.

Important notes:

The fish oil should ideally be at a ratio of 2:1 DHA to EPA – and our patients are still required to take a fish oil supplement as well. MCT oil could also be a good option. Some preliminary research shows it's good for sperm health as well as gut and metabolic health.[10,11] A combination of MCT and DHA containing fish oils in the lemon drink can be ideal if dealing with egg-quality and/or sperm-quality issues. Alternatively, you can use coconut butter (there are many recipes online if you want to make your own). I recommend cycling your fats and using different ones from time to time, as it ensures your body gets a varied fatty-acid profile, which is ideal for optimum health.

Do not use soy or soya-based lecithin. You may omit the lecithin if you wish, but it's best to try and find the right lecithin, if possible.

You can use a 1000-IU strength vitamin E capsule if you've never had rheumatic fever – buy a good-quality brand that doesn't include soy as an ingredient or excipient. One week before or after an egg pickup, you may wish to omit the vitamin E.

The whole lemon drink can be safely consumed throughout your reproductive cycle and pregnancy, and it's also fine to consume during an IVF cycle because ultimately it constitutes a food – not a supplement.

When storing the drink, ensure the glass container is as full as possible to decrease the amount of air within the container (air speeds up oxidation). And be sure to increase your intake of plain *filtered* water to two to three litres daily to aid in optimal cellular function.

Fertility Reset Prescription 2: Enjoy the whole lemon drink elixir

Your task for today is to make yourself the ultimate fertility mocktail: the whole lemon drink. Enjoy it with your partner.

Resources

If you have questions about the whole lemon drink, or if you want to see me making it in my own kitchen, visit the Fertility Breakthrough interactive book portal at http://thefertile.me/BreakthroughBook.

References

1 Albert, S.M., et al., Promoting safe and effective use of OTC medications: CHPA-GSA National Summit. *The Gerontologist*, 2014. 54(6).

2 Jackowski, S.A., et al., Oxidation levels of North American over-the-counter n-3 (omega-3) supplements and the influence of supplement formulation and delivery form on evaluating oxidative safety. *Journal of Nutritional Science*, 2015. 4.

3 Mohseni, M., et al., Prevalence and reasons of self-medication in pregnant women: A systematic review and meta-analysis. *International Journal of Community Based Nursing and Midwifery*, 2018. 6(4).

4 Birkhäuer, J., et al., Trust in the health care professional and health outcome: A meta-analysis. *PLoS One*, 2017. 12(2).

5 Mathur, S., et al., Personalized medicine could transform healthcare. *Biomedical Reports*, 2017. 7(1).

6 Kelley, K.E., et al., Identification of phthalates in medications and dietary supplement formulations in the United States and Canada. *Environmental Health Perspectives*, 2012. 120(3).

7 Kumar, A., et al., The mystery ingredients: Sweeteners, flavorings, dyes, and preservatives in analgesic/antipyretic, antihistamine/decongestant, cough and cold, antidiarrheal, and liquid theophylline preparations. *Pediatrics*, 1993. 91(5).

8 Napke, E., et al., Excipients and additives: Hidden hazards in drug products and in product substitution. *Canadian Medical Association Journal*, 1984. 131(12).

9 What are excipients doing in medicinal products? *Drugs and Therapeutics Bulletin*, 2009. 47(7).

10 Kim, N., et al., Effect of lipid metabolism on male fertility. *Biochemical and Biophysical Research Communications*, 2017. 485(3).

11 Rial, S.A., et al., Gut microbiota and metabolic health: The potential beneficial effects of a medium chain triglyceride diet in obese individuals. *Nutrients*, 2016. 8(5).

CHAPTER 10

Prescription 3: Protect Your Relationship From The Stresses Of Infertility And Miscarriage

'Happy couples understand that helping each other realise their dreams is one of the goals of marriage.'

Dr John Gottman

I value family greatly, so it's no surprise I've found myself helping to create families for the last two decades. A solid and robust family environment begins before a baby enters the picture. It all starts with a strong tribe. If you're courageously embarking on the path of solo reproduction, you likely have people in your life to whom you can apply the concepts I'll discuss next.

Your relationship with your partner matters. In a relationship, two people get to share life's load, but two people also need to sort through the inevitable challenges and ups and downs, and a difficult fertility journey adds further pressure.

Let's face it: if you've chosen to have a child with someone, your relationship is critical to your fertility success. You need a sense of equanimity through the inevitably troubling times; supporting and being supported by your partner needs to be a priority. Either partner's neglect of the critical fact that good relationships are created and don't just happen will break your bond as a couple. You will begin turning away from rather than towards each other for support and this starts to spell the beginning of the end of otherwise potentially great relationships. In this section, I want to help you discover ways to navigate the rocky times and make it all work, for you both.[1,2] But know this very clearly: infertility cannot destroy your relationship, just as a baby cannot save it. The responsibility for your own happiness is solely yours – nobody else's. Not even if you choose to share your life with another.

Being a wonderful partner (like being a great parent) requires giving of yourself, especially when you don't want to or you don't feel like it. When times are tough, you need to remind yourself that the only thing you can control is what *you* do, think and therefore feel. And I do mean remind *yourself* – not your partner. The only thing 'nagging' is good for is getting your partner offside and guaranteeing you'll have more of what you don't want in your relationship. On the flip side, if you happen to be the person repeatedly being 'reminded' of something, you need to understand that only when you choose to alter your behaviour and do things differently will you receive a gentler, kinder and more loving response. If you expect the other person to change so you can be happy, you'll be forever unfulfilled – no matter which side of that equation you find yourself on. As Gandhi said, 'Be the change you want to see in the world', and what a better place to start than in your relationship.

For a relationship to work, two people must be willing to consistently bring the best of themselves to each encounter. And although your best will vary from time to time, the key is to bring everything you can. Each partner must bring 100% of themselves and their effort for the sake of the whole. Why? Simple multiplication. If you bring only 50% of your A game and your partner brings only 50%, you both end up with a quarter of the whole. If you bring your 50% and your partner brings 100%, you still have only 50% of everything you could – ultimately bringing the team down. When you and your partner each bring your version of 100% in as many situations as you possibly can, then and only then do you have a chance of ending up with an infinitely better situation – the complete, encouraging and loving relationship you deserve.

Have you ever got upset because your partner isn't always supportive, happy, giving, kind and loving? Because you're met with challenge, unhappiness, selfishness and lack of support? It's simply not possible for a relationship to be perfect. It's important to realise that most people's idea of a great relationship is a fantasy.

• MUM KNOWS BEST •

My mum, a practical and smart lady, always said, 'Relationships only change house numbers.' And I can attest to that because before I married the amazing man who is the father of my children, I was married to an equally great person. So, what went wrong? For starters, we were young, and it turned out we wanted different things out of life. And I hadn't internalised this concept that relationships only change 'location'. I hadn't yet fully recognised the degree to which the lessons I needed to learn would keep showing up (through different people) in very similar ways until I learned them. After all, I was the common denominator in all my relationships. So, after the initial honeymoon period of a new relationship, I found myself having similar frustrations in my next relationship.

But these were very different men. My first husband was about my age. My second (and current) husband was ten years my senior – a solid, kind and experienced man. Yet, the nit-picking that had driven me crazy before was happening all over again, and in one of those 'why-the-hell-am-I-in-this-relationship-with-this-most-annoying-person-in-the-world' moments (because clearly I'm the perfect one, right?) it hit me like a flash of lightning: 'What am I doing to this poor man to elicit the exact same behaviour I despised in my last relationship and didn't want to experience in this relationship?'

And that was the first time I really understood the concept that the response I get is utterly and completely a result of whom I choose to be and how *I act* in any given moment. There was no point blaming my partner for how annoying 'he was' if I wasn't willing to take full responsibility and play above the line in my relationship. It was here I truly consolidated the learning that for things 'out there' to change, first, I must change.

The concept of playing above the line was extremely powerful for me. I had it on the door of my fridge for many years, until I fully internalised it.

This is something you can easily visualise. Draw a line in the centre of a piece of paper. Below the line lives the victim who blames, denies and makes excuses. Above the line lives the victor who revels in taking ownership, being accountable and taking personal responsibility. Ask yourself these questions when thinking about your relationship: Where am I playing right now? Where have I been playing for a while? Above the line or below the line? Sure, we might all dip below that imaginary (yet very real) line from time to time, but if you're living below the line, you're short-changing yourself and the people you love. And unless you have a real plan to get out of there fast, you're inevitably digging your relationship's grave.

ACCOUNTABILITY ◆	PERSONAL RESPONSIBILITY	◆ OWNERSHIP

I am committed   I want to understand   I DO   X,Y,Z   I choose to bring my "A" game

I choose to learn   I #GSD!   I AM   FINDING A   I am grateful   I give my 100%

I AM IN CONTROL   BETTER

↑ ABOVE THE LINE   I am hopeful WAY   I AM TAKING ACTION

It's too hard   I WAS TOLD   you always do this   I'M TOO TIRED   I am waiting   BELOW THE LINE ↓

I CAN'T BE BOTHERED   you said for...

THERE IS NOTHING I CAN DO   It's not my fault   that's because X.Y.Z happened   It's their fault   I SHOULDN'T HAVE TO DO THIS

I give up   IT'S NOT MY JOB   Why me?

BLAME ◆	EXCUSE ◆	DENIAL

• ARE YOU PLAYING ABOVE THE LINE? •

How can you figure out where you're playing most of the time? It's simple – answer these questions:

- Do you feel like your partner is constantly nagging you?

Or could it be that you're consistently behaving like a child who needs to be reminded of things?

- Do you feel like the person you're with is too inflexible and wants everything their own way?

Or is it that you're holding your position like a stubborn mule, constantly making the same mistakes or excuses for yourself?

- Do you blame your partner for never following through with commitments you make as a couple regarding working on and improving your relationship?

Or is it that you're expecting they take responsibility for making your relationship better while you get away with not consistently bringing and/or doing your best?

It's an immutable fact that for things 'out there' to change, things inside you must change first. There are two sides to everything. You must recognise that you're the only one who can take ownership for the health of your relationship. You're the only one who can take responsibility for making it the best it can be. Embody and enact the change you want to see – permanently. Otherwise, nothing will ever change. Of course, some relationships aren't right, and if that's where you are, you need to rise above the line and ask yourself:

'What is the first step I need to take to stop wasting my time here?' If you don't want to leave, then commit to making the relationship the very best it can be.

This applies to you. Don't think this is some random message meant for some other person. I don't believe in random, or that things just happen for no reason. There is huge, deep learning in what you're experiencing right now in the guise of infertility (or recurrent miscarriage). Perhaps you think your reproductive challenges are destroying your relationship, self-confidence and self-love. But can we be courageous, get real for a moment, as difficult as this may feel? You're the only one who has the power to change your beliefs, which in turn leads to a change in your thinking, which leads to new actions and, finally, different results. Implementing this understanding is the best way to create lasting change. Your job is to immerse yourself in this concept and let it percolate just enough so you can take action on it quickly. As if your happiness depends on it. Because it does.

MIRACLE MOMENTS

• NOT LONELY AND ISOLATED •
ALISON AND PHIL

My husband and I had a son together, and then we decided that we would like to add to our family. I'd always dreamt of quite a large family – I wanted five children. So, we started trying, and nothing happened straightaway. I wasn't particularly concerned or worried, but after about a year, I felt that perhaps I should go and see a doctor about it. Though, because I was in my late twenties and my husband was young too, the doctor simply told us not to worry about it and that it would be fine.

We persisted but still nothing happened, so the doctor sent us off for some initial tests, which all came back fine. We were then referred to a fertility specialist, who also did more testing. Left feeling personally and emotionally violated after many invasive tests and procedures, we were then given the mystifying diagnosis of 'unexplained infertility'. They couldn't find anything wrong and had no idea why we were having difficulties.

We were healthy. We both exercised several times during the week. We were non-smokers. We were also very moderate with our caffeine intake, and by this time, I was completely off alcohol and my husband very infrequently had a drink. Our diet was healthy, with meat and lots of vegetables. I was particularly careful about the use of pesticides and chemicals around our house. We kept on seeing a fertility specialist for a number of years, and at the same time I also explored alternative therapies, such as acupuncture and herbal treatments.

Our four-year journey had taken a toll on us financially. Fertility treatment is very expensive. But worse were the emotional costs. We'd had a son with no problems whatsoever, and we were doing 'everything right'. I'd had online consultations with fertility specialists in the USA, and frankly felt ripped off. I'd bought books on the internet hoping for the miracles they promised, and still nothing had helped.

I said to my husband, 'I can't do this anymore. I can't keep fighting the system asking for answers. I need an advocate. I need someone to put it all together for me.' It was then that I stumbled upon Gabriela. From our first conversation she was confident and knowledgeable, and her belief and energy were contagious, so we invited her to come on board as a partner with us during our journey to try to create ourselves a healthy baby and a larger family.

I'm sure that like me, many women on their fertility journey can sometimes feel a bit lonely and isolated, and the emotions that you feel can often be quite different from what your partner feels. The thing I loved most about Gabriela's Natural Fertility Breakthrough Program™ was the structured support. Although I have a lovely and supportive husband, it was really useful that we had to meet together at each session to learn things together. We had homework that we got to do together, and we worked through so much (physically, environmentally and emotionally). It helped to keep him on track and involved.

After the initial 120-day preparation stage, I still wasn't pregnant. Other people on the program were celebrating their positive results. But not us. After a while, Gabriela suggested we change conception strategies and give IVF a chance, but I just wasn't ready emotionally. I explained how I felt and that I wanted to continue trying naturally.

Gabriela supported our decision and helped us continue doing all the best things for our bodies. She kept us going – always making improvements along the way. Then, seemingly out of the blue, we got a positive pregnancy test! For so long, I'd been in the infertility mindset, and all of a sudden, we were pregnant. It was so exciting. We had our beautiful girl. We then revisited the program and this time very quickly had a boy, followed by another blissful boy. We have been incredibly blessed with three #TEAMROSA babies. Life now is deliciously full with our four children. Hubby says it's enough! I feel incredibly blessed to have found Gabriela.

You can graduate to the next level in your relationship, but make no mistake – you're never done. There will always be the next challenge to work through and overcome along with the permanent ones you learn to manage and navigate. That's the nature of being human, of evolving. We grow on the precipice of challenge and support. Life is a combination of good and bad, so quit wasting your life looking for the relationship that's always perfect. It doesn't exist.

Your choice is plain and simple – make what you've got the masterpiece it has the potential to be, the masterpiece you deserve, irrespective of its quirks and imperfections. Or find a place where there are no other humans and you can exist alone (though I'll hazard a guess that inner turmoil will resurface sooner or later, despite the initial peace and quiet). If these words resonate and you've started to berate yourself, let me ask you this: Where are you playing right now? Above or below the line? Quit trying to be perfect and take ownership of simply doing your best. Whenever you fail, acknowledge it, know that it was your best at the time, resolve to do better next time, and move on.

So how does this apply to your fertility? It's simple: if your partner has had to 'nag' (aka make a reasonable request of you, multiple times) you to get involved, to do your part, to give it your best to optimise your fertility for the sake of you and your family, frankly, they deserve better and so do you. And remember, talk is cheap. If you're constantly talking about how much you want a baby and your actions demonstrate a completely different set of values, desires and actions, then take responsibility.

Discomfort, in any endeavour, is a reasonably reliable indicator that growth is required. Whenever you feel that something external is forcing you to do something you don't particularly want to do (but is for your ultimate benefit and will improve your well-being), recognise that 'growing' awaits, and sometimes growing pains are very real. There's always a choice, and the best choice is to play above the line, not below it.

This is your moment. If there are conversations you need to have and decisions you need to make, do these things now. It will never get easier, and time will pass. Leave it too long and you may run out of time altogether. The time to clear the air and realign your commitment to yourself, to your relationship and to your dreams is *now*.

Finally, it's important to acknowledge that you and your partner may need different things from each other in order to feel loved. You need to know or perhaps even rediscover your wants and needs as they relate to your partner and your relationship. In turn, you may need to discover or rediscover your partner's.

Neither of you is the same as you were when you first met, so updating your 'love maps' (an idea developed by world-renowned relationship researcher Dr John Gottman) is essential if you want a relationship that keeps on growing and thriving as the years pass.[9] It's utterly possible to have a deeply connected, loving and evolving relationship despite the challenges you endure together, including infertility and miscarriage. A little tender loving care, a mountain of kindness and empathy with an extra special dash of patience will be required.

The beautiful orange daisies that blossom and multiply each year through the cracks in my concrete driveway (despite the thoroughfare traffic) remind me daily that strong desire coupled with determined action is what gets you what you want. Assuming you've decided that your relationship is worth the effort (remember, every relationship requires your devoted energy), then applied persistence is what will take the relationship to the level you desire.

MIRACLE MOMENTS

• MAKE THE SMALL MOMENTS PRECIOUS •
NATALIA AND MIRO

My husband, Miro, and I were 31 and 33 respectively when we were due to get married, and we knew we wanted babies as soon as possible. We were no strangers to natural health. We ate home-cooked whole foods, we'd been purchasing organic food and home products for ten years and were fit and exercised regularly. At the time my job was stressful and I also decided to make a career change and started studying Traditional Chinese Medicine.

About five months before our wedding, we started our pre-conception preparation. I tracked my basal body temperature and cycles and started seeing a Chinese medicine practitioner – and after over a year of doing all of that, there was still no baby. So, we began searching further and wider. Our standard GP tests showed there was nothing wrong, so I began seeing an ever-growing list of practitioners: different Chinese medicine practitioners, a chiropractor and an osteopath; I also went for massages and acupuncture regularly, and did yoga. I researched as much as I could find to uncover answers or another path that could help us.

I began to feel more despairing. I couldn't understand why I was doing everything I knew and that I could – and still nothing was working! I was tired and felt completely worn out.

Trying each month and then getting my period was distressing and constantly weighed on my mind. One thing I knew for sure: I wasn't ready to give up. But I was exhausted and getting nowhere.

Fortunately, our relationship was strong. Miro was amazing at helping me shift my frame of mind. Our best relationship saver was making small moments precious. We'd catch each other passing in the hallway and share a brief but truly intimate kiss, or stop mid-conversation and really look at each other and say, 'I love you', or, 'Thank you for being you'. Sex was, however, becoming a task and lacking spark and spontaneity. It became really difficult to connect on that level.

It was at the peak of my despair, when we finally found Gabriela. I was drawn to the thoroughness of her program and the fact that it encompassed everything in our lives. It took our whole picture into consideration, not just 'my' or 'our' fertility. I felt like I'd finally found someone who was different from other practitioners I'd seen.

As we read through the material and started the program, I was happy we were turning over each stone and that we were leaving nothing to chance. Looking back now, I recognise that the things that were truly in our way were the things we didn't even know we didn't know at the time, just as Gabriela had told us. We learned the importance of minor factors when it comes to fertility and how they compound to create one big lack of results.

I felt a complete sense of relief and well-founded hope when I started on the Natural Fertility Breakthrough Program™. We finally had a purpose and we threw ourselves into the details.

I won't lie – at first, it was hard work. There were so many new things to learn and factor into our lives, but at the same time, it was refreshing to be taking charge of my results

After a few months we started to feel better with all the changes we were making. We had more energy and our bodies seemed to be responding to everything well, plus our test results were improving. This time of preparation, where we weren't actively trying to conceive, was actually a huge relief – but it also didn't feel like we were wasting time at all because we had absolute clarity about what we were working on and what we needed to create to make it all happen.

After our initial period of preparation, I was pregnant within three cycles. I was elated! Our treatment and Gabriela's support continued throughout what was a very easy pregnancy, helping me support my body and growing baby as well as preparation for a healthy birth.

My little miracle, Eliana, arrived in a peaceful and entirely natural water-birth delivery. Eliana is now almost four, and she continues to be a strong, robust, amazing little girl, having had nothing more than a minor cold in her entire life!

And the story of course didn't end there. Because of how long it took us to conceive Eliana, we thought we would start our preparation early for baby number two. We knew we wanted to have more children, and knowing we couldn't take our fertility and the precious gift of children for granted, when Eliana was about nine months old and my period returned, we came back to revisit Gabriela's program and our preconception preparation again.

My pregnancy had been so great but it was highly taxing on my body's nutrient levels. And the new baby changed many things about our lifestyle; the sleep deprivation that came with it also added a level of intensity that wasn't previously there.

We also knew that our current medical status had to be considered and looked at with fresh eyes. This time, everything we were doing to optimise our health and fertility just felt like a natural part of life, and after our preconception phase we conceived easily and naturally after a few cycles. We were totally amazed.

Unfortunately, our joy was short-lived when I miscarried at seven and a half weeks. I felt my body just wasn't yet ready. Our despair was enormous. Gabriela reassured us, and we buckled down again and reassessed what was going on. We revised our treatments and continued our journey.

It took me a long time to process the grief, and energetically, I think I was trying to get that baby back rather than letting go, accepting that it wasn't their time. I was so very blessed to already have Eliana. She was my light helping me through and making me smile when I was down. My shift came when I was truly able to let go. I spent more time being kind to myself and forgiving myself for the miscarriage, even though intellectually I knew it wasn't my fault. I distinctly remember the moment I was able to grieve: properly grieve. I got pregnant with our next child one week after that! Exactly one year and one week after our last bub.

This pregnancy also went smoothly. Jakub was born in a beautiful natural, home water birth, at a whopping, healthy 4.5 kilograms. Eliana was there the whole time and shared this precious day with us.

It's important to build upon and strengthen the *friendship* in your romantic relationship. Friendship is the foundation of a happy and loving union, at whatever stage you find yourself in. In fact, relationship research shows that strong relationships are built on great friendship.[3,4,5] Think about this for a moment. Imagine you have a friend who lives in a different city, so you don't see each other often, and they're coming to visit you. It's a big, exciting occasion and you want to make the two weeks you'll spend together special and unforgettable for you both.

Now let's say things don't go exactly to plan during their stay. How do you choose to spend your time? Do you sulk because they don't do exactly what you want? Do you decide to be inflexible about where to go? Of course not – you make concessions. Above all, you're interested in what's happening in their world. You ask questions about what's been happening in their life, and you're genuinely interested in hearing their thoughts on all sorts of things. You want to know about their hopes and aspirations for the visit and beyond. You check in with how they're feeling – Are they enjoying themselves? What's their mood? Would they prefer to do something different? And you don't take their responses personally. In short, you make the space and time, you turn towards them (physically and metaphorically) and you connect. Your friend is enveloped in your pleasant warmth and as a result responds in kind. The outcome is that you both enjoy yourselves and strengthen your friendship bond. Your friendship account is topped up, and when you're apart again, you remember with fondness your time together. You note you even navigated minor or major annoyances pretty well because you applied curiosity to understanding how they arose. You both chose not to 'sweat the small stuff'. In the overall balance, you were both courteous, kind, considerate of each other's feelings.

It doesn't take any more than this to have a brilliant romantic relationship. This kind of loving and connected friendship is the essential ingredient of the relationship you, your partner and your future family deserve.[6,7]

Fertility Reset Prescription 3: More than words

It's always nice to also hear 'I love you', but the bottom line is that being shown has a longer-lasting effect. [8,9]

When it comes to showing your partner how you feel, the first step is to take full responsibility and consciously act (at least most of the time) in accordance with the response you want to receive from your partner. Some people think that 'if my partner really loves me, then it's their problem and responsibility to deal with my garbage'. Wrong. The best relationships are based on solid foundations of mutual and self-respect. You know that if you consistently treat your friends badly, if they have any self-respect, in time they are not going to stand for it. Why should your partner? And even if you stay together out of a sense of obligation, you will both pay the price in miserable co-existence. So remember, your partner will eventually respond in kind. Even if at the outset that desired response is delayed, remain steadfast and remember, there will be a little retraining required. Your own positive and consistent action will eventually create a positive reserve in your relationship bank account, which has perhaps been overdrawn for some time. So, keep at it. If you continue to act as if you want to be your partner's best friend, consistently, it's only a matter of time until you both create the relationship you deserve. [10,11,12]

How can you begin this relationship reinvention? Start with the little things. Play games that make you both laugh; let them know why you think they're great at their job; do a load of washing from beginning to end without having to be asked; write them a love letter; empty the dishwasher; give them a foot massage; cook their favourite meal, serve a tropical fruit platter for dessert wearing only your sexiest smile; let them pick the next movie you watch together; take them out on a picnic at sunrise; finally give in and sign up for that dance class they've been wanting you to accompany them to for years, even though you think you'd rather not. You know? Deep down, you already know what you need to do.

But if you think you don't know, or need reminding, then this is your task. Ask your partner to compile a list of fifty things that make them feel loved, romanced and cared for – the small, the big and the tiny. You do the same, and then swap lists. You'll have so many laughs chatting about and exploring what made it onto those lists, and you'll have plenty of ideas to implement. Most importantly, have fun in the process.

Resources

If you're unsure whether you want to stay in a relationship, be sure to read and do the exercises in the book *Too Good to Leave, Too Bad to Stay*, by Mira Kirshenbaum. It's a must read if you want to make a conscious and deliberate decision that will be best for you and your partner in the long term.

And in the interactive portal for this book, I've included some additional resources to help you begin creating the solid foundation your relationship deserves. You'll find educational resources and books I recommend to my patients, who go on to create thriving relationships and much more. Simply visit http://thefertile.me/ BreakthroughBook for access.

References

1   Gottman, J.M., et al., Marital interaction and satisfaction: A longitudinal view. *Journal of Consulting and Clinical Psychology*, 1989. 57(1).

2   Shapiro, A.F., et al., Short-term change in couples' conflict following a transition to parenthood intervention. *Couple & Family Psychology*, 2015. 4(4).

3   Grote, N.K., et al., The measurement of Friendship-based Love in intimate relationships. *Personal Relationships*, 1994. 1(3).

4   Hecht, M.L., et al., Love ways and relationship quality in heterosexual relationships. *Journal of Social and Personal Relationships*, 1994. 11(1).

5   VanderDrift, L.E., et al., On the benefits of valuing being friends for nonmarital romantic partners. *Journal of Social and Personal Relationships*, 2013. 30(1).

6   Cleary Bradley, R.P., et al., Reducing situational violence in low-income couples by fostering healthy relationships. *Journal of Marital and Family Therapy*, 2012. 38 (Suppl 1).

7   Gottman, J.M., et al., The effects of briefly interrupting marital conflict. *Journal of Marital and Family Therapy*, 2018. 44(1).

8   Davoodvandi, M., et al., Examining the effectiveness of Gottman couple therapy on improving marital adjustment and couples' intimacy. *Iranian Journal of Psychiatry*, 2018. 13(2).

9   Gottman, J., et al., *The Seven Principles for Making Marriage Work*. 1999, London, UK: Orion Books.

10   Kogan, A., et al., When giving feels good. The intrinsic benefits of sacrifice in romantic relationships for the communally motivated. *Psychological Science*, 2010. 21(12).

11   Le, B.M., et al., Communal motivation and well-being in interpersonal relationships: An integrative review and meta-analysis. *Psychological Bulletin*, 2018. 144(1).

12   Madhyastha, T.M., et al., Investigating spousal influence using moment-to-moment affect data from marital conflict. *Journal of Family Psychology: JFP*: Journal of the Division of Family Psychology of the American Psychological Association (Division 43), 2011. 25(2).

CHAPTER 11

Prescription 4: The Mindset Of Creating Positive Fertility Change

M any times in life you have to say no to the things you want most in favour of the things you want more.

Within three days of consumption, everything we eat and drink has been assimilated into our bodies and has become part of the cells within our system. Food is the cement that keeps us together, alive and (depending on our choices) well. It's also what our bodies use when repairs and maintenance are required and when we need to build new cells. In the first instance (derived from a myriad of interdependent biological processes), healthy sperm and eggs – which later become a brand-new healthy baby – have their humble origins in the building blocks found in food.

With so many food fads and dieting trends telling us what (or not) to eat, it's no wonder there's so much confusion about what helps humans thrive. But eating for health and reproductive balance is simple. Fresh, unprocessed and organic/biodynamic foods – a diet predominantly based on vegetables, good-quality animal protein and healthy fats (with a little 10% for the soul, from time to time) – are the best sources of complete nutrients for optimum fertility.[1,2,3,4,5,6,7,8,9,10,11,12,13]

Overall, most people have a pretty good concept of what healthy eating looks like. However, when it comes to the crunch (pun intended), we often end up making not-so-healthy choices. We could blame the whole universe for this, but the reason we make unhealthy choices arises from a much more practical consideration: essentially, we believe there's more pleasure (even if fleeting) in eating that piece of fried chicken or donut than there is pain – despite the fact that in time, the negative consequences of our poor choices are often irreversibly severe and long lasting.[14,15] You would choose the steamed vegetables and grilled organic chicken (despite the higher cost and perhaps more restricted availability) if you, overall, understood and agreed that the benefits of eating this way far outweighed the drawbacks (which they do), and if you were also consciously invested in this idea.[16,17,18,19]

In many countries around the world, people make better food choices not based on availability but on education and, even more so, on a shift in beliefs and mindset.[20,21,22,23] This truth is abundantly clear within cultures where most people's basic needs are already met. As humans, we prioritise and will even sacrifice ourselves in pursuit of making happen what we value most.[24,25] However, my patients have taught me that deeply connecting with and reinforcing the why of a certain behaviour is the key to creating long-lasting change. As a result of my clinical observations over the years, I've concluded that the greatest difficulty most people have in making the required changes in this area and, even more importantly, in making those changes last, comes from identifying the specific and effective tools and strategies that can help them arrive at the right mindset – the mindset required to make new and improved daily choices out of habit. But I've also seen that when these important links are firmly in place, seemingly miraculous changes in behaviour are possible. The fact that you have this book in your hands puts you in a privileged position indeed. You can implement what I've learned through decades of observation, trial and error, and you can use it to your benefit right now.

To help my patients make changes (which include lifestyle and habit modifications), I created a three-step process that amalgamates various tried and tested tools to enable long-lasting habit change. In this instance, we're using it to address lifestyle behaviour. But you can use it for anything you want to let go of that no longer serves you (stress, anxiety, worry, addictions and more). I call it the Life Changer Method™. Starting afresh in any area of your life is as simple as these three steps: first you *face it*, then you *feel it*, so you can *flow with it*. I've organised these steps based on neuroscience and mindfulness research and have successfully applied the method with thousands of patients over the years. An unsolicited word of caution here, though: just reading about this methodology won't change your life any more than medicine left in a bottle would. You need to implement what you learn consistently. You need to transform in a way that leads to the results you're looking for in your life.

I believe you can. Now, the *choice* is yours.

The Life Changer Method™ deconstructed

Sometimes we need to break things down before we can break through, so let's begin.

Step 1 – Face it

Clarity is everything. Facing the things we perceive as difficult isn't exactly a part of the 'pleasure seeking and pain avoiding' human DNA that sees discomfort as a threat to survival. As a result of this evolutionary fact, we often hand over our power and seek to avoid all that's 'uncomfortable' because, what if that big scary monster were to gobble us up? It is now a childish explanation for a behaviour that for millions of years kept us safe. Despite its previous benefits, turning away from discomfort as if it were a life-threatening danger is for the most part an ineffective strategy.

Carl Jung said, 'What we resist persists.' Think about it. The more you try to fight something – a craving, a dissatisfaction, a fear – the more it grows and occupies your awareness. It takes root in your heart and mind.

So much of our anxiety is about the imagined worst-case scenario of a given situation rather about what's actually happening. Whenever I was in the throes of imagined despair as a dramatic teenager, my dad would say to me, 'Don't suffer in anticipation.' I've grown to see this as sage advice. But for a long time, I wondered, 'How do you *not* suffer in anticipation?'

One day the answer came to me: you do your best. Not more or less than your best. Your best. Without trying to control the outcome. Without deciding that you can only be happy if things turn out in the exact way you envision in your mind. You open yourself up to a wisdom greater than your own by simply doing your best.

The first step in facing anything is accepting it, acknowledging it's there. You don't have to like it. You just need to objectively surrender. No matter how scared you are about this step, I promise you: the *doing* of it is easier than you might *think*. The thinking (or more accurately, the imagining of the unknown and the scary consequences arising from what is) is the part that gets in the way of accepting.

So take the emotion out of it. There's nothing wrong with any particular situation – the meaning we choose to embed in it is what creates our experience of it. When you choose to face something, your purpose isn't to label it or give it meaning (eg 'I'm such a loser because I keep eating sugar when I know I shouldn't'). You're simply meant to see it for what it is (eg 'I keep eating junk food and I know this isn't helping me achieve what I want. This is something I'd like to change'). The first statement puts you down; the second puts you in charge – and that's exactly where you belong (and the only place from which you can change anything). It doesn't matter that you might not yet know how to change the issue you're facing. You just need to acknowledge that it's no longer serving you and that you want to do something about it.

Facing it puts you above the line – your place of power.

When people place their unrelenting focus on the ultimate thing they cannot control on their fertility journey (ie having a baby), much unhappiness ensues. Let's face this together: trying to control the outcome of having a baby is as effective as trying to control the weather to stop the rain. It's impossible. Besides, what's wrong with the rain anyway? It provides a pattern interrupt, an opportunity to see things from a different perspective (just like the fertility journey *wink wink*).

What you can control is your response to the rain – you can allow yourself more time to get to places; you can wear boots and a raincoat; you can carry an umbrella or maybe even a change of clothes in a water-resistant bag. And when it comes to having a baby, you can adopt a healthier diet, make better lifestyle choices and reduce your exposure to chemicals within your personal environment to positively influence or even remove obstacles and minor factors present in your situation and optimise your fertility.

The key to overcoming fertility problems (and miscarriage) is to gather all the scattered 'puzzle pieces' and determine where you can and need to intervene and what you simply cannot control. It will never be your job to control a baby's development in utero. It will be your job to feed yourself and the baby the right nutrients. Your behaviour associated with having a healthy diet (and everything else I discuss in this book and beyond) is all you can and need to influence.

So use your energy wisely. Focus on doing your best in the areas in which you want to see change – for the highest good of all concerned. It's that simple.

• BEHAVIOUR, NOT RESULTS •

Author Jim Camp says, 'By following your behavioral goals, you get your objectives. Instead of trying to break par, a result we cannot control, we concentrate on putting a good swing on the ball, an action we can control. What you can control is behaviour and activity. What you cannot control is the result of this behaviour and activity. Think behaviour, forget results.' Results are a direct consequence of a correct strategy coupled with the right behaviour and activity.

In the context of improving your diet (remember, you can use the Life Changer Method™ in any area of your life), the first step is to get clear on the *one* thing[26] you can do that will make everything else easier or unnecessary.

For example, you might have identified that you end up giving in to sugary snacks in the afternoon or evening because you're skipping meals or aren't eating enough protein at breakfast. Upon further self-inquiry, you identify this is happening because you don't have the ingredients in the house to prepare adequate meals and you don't have the ability to get them at the last minute. As a result, you see that not having a weekly meal plan from which you can derive an appropriate shopping list is a problem you need to resolve.

This entire chain of thinking happened as quickly as asking yourself this critical clarifying question: What's the one thing I can do to improve my diet in a way that will make everything else easier or unnecessary?

Finally, note that the question isn't 'What are the top five things I can do?' but rather 'What is the *one* thing I can do?' This is very important. You need to focus and drill into what's the most important. There may be many useful things you can do, but one will make everything else easier or unnecessary first. Once that's in place, you can ask again and focus on improving, fine tuning and optimising.

The first step in the Life Changer Method™ may well be enough to change 'surface issues'. Now it's time for the next step.

Step 2 – Feel it

This step is an exercise in contrast which leverages what the human psyche prizes most: moving away from pain and towards pleasure.

It quickly connects you to why change is a must now and not 'one day'. The purpose of this step is to link together all the costs of not changing now (aka the pain) and to understand how you will benefit when you do (towards pleasure).

By now you will have identified a dietary or lifestyle habit you'd like to modify (*face it*). Always think in terms of an action or inaction on your part rather than in terms of something that you perceive is being done 'to' you. Because even if the perception feels true, at some level, there will be an action or inaction on your part making the situation possible.

Pick something you've been stuck on that you haven't been able to shift in the past (due to your own action or inaction) and that causes you (real or perceived) pain. This issue will be what you set out to straighten in the *feel it* step, right now.

Your job is to answer four questions on paper.[27] Writing is the 'doing' part of thinking and connecting new neuropathways.[28,29] Plan to use at least one to three double-sided sheets for each question. Aim to come up with at least thirty to fifty answers to each one of the example questions below (it's easy to come up with even more because for each thing you list, several other elements might spring to mind. To elicit and become aware of other facets of the problem, with each cost you write down ask yourself: 'Why is this a problem?').

You'll need to set aside one or two hours to complete this exercise (gadgets off and stowed away). Gather water, paper, pens, tissues and whatever else you need so you don't have to search for things while completing this exercise. To do this properly, you need to have no interruptions. And I promise that when you're done, you'll *know*. You'll feel it in every fibre of your being and you'll be able to implement whatever it is you're choosing to do differently with incredible ease.

Let's begin.

Question one: What is it costing me right now (physically, emotionally, financially, spiritually, relationship-wise and in every other way) to *indulge in the need to eat damaging junk food*?

You can change the italicised sentenced above to anything you want to address, in any area of your life, from smoking to drinking coffee or alcohol to laziness at work to hitting the snooze button too many times – any habit or behaviour you engage in that doesn't positively serve you and that you'd like to change. You just need to be very specific and choose something that's a result of a clear action or inaction on your part.

The first time I used this exercise, I wanted to stop eating chocolate. I had a serious chocolate addiction ('addiction' defined as continued use or engagement with the behaviour, despite adverse consequences). Given that I'd been diagnosed with PCOS and wanted to regulate my cycle, there were decidedly many adverse consequences to continuing to indulge in chocolate. I was berating myself for not 'being able' to stop and constantly feeling bad that I was fighting this 'losing battle' and getting down on myself as a result (I didn't understand the *face it* step then). It was an infuriating and self-defeating cycle. Enough was enough. I had arrived at the point where change became a must. I applied this exercise to the point of sobbing tears – and it's still the most remarkably cathartic experience I've ever had. It showed me the power of linking up the costs and really *feeling* them rather than just intellectualising them or trying (and ultimately failing) to explain them away and wishing I'd 'feel better'. When I was done, I had broken the addiction. For five years after, I didn't even want to get near chocolate. Today, some eight years on, chocolate remains where it belonged all along, in the 'take it or leave it' basket. Pleasurable yes, but no longer the obsession it was. Such a liberating exercise.

So, get clear and decide what you want to address. As you go along, you can dig deeper by asking yourself: 'What else is it costing me?' 'How else is it costing me?' 'Who else is being hurt or even damaged, today or in the future, by my continuing to do this?' When you feel you're running out of things to write down (the well is deep, be sure to empty it out completely), link as much pain and suffering to the behaviour you want to change as possible. Also be sure to involve as many areas of your life as possible in your answers. Only in doing so do you create enough leverage over yourself to enable deep and lasting cognitive restructuring (aka change).[30,31,32] This step facilitates enough distance from your addiction to allow you to break the romanticised infatuation with the perceived benefits of the behaviour. Once you've squeezed every last cost onto paper, move on to question two. But be sure to add anything to any section that may come to mind while you're doing another part of this step. If you think it, it should go down on paper. The more you bring these thoughts, feelings and ideas to the light, facing and feeling them, the easier they are to let go.

• DEEP-DIVING: A WAY OF VISUALISING THIS PROCESS •

Here's an example from a conversation I once had with one of my patients:

'Indulging in sugary treats and drinks is causing me to be overweight. This is causing problems in my relationship.'

Why is that a problem?
It makes me feel unattractive and retreat within myself.

Why is that a problem?
It disconnects me from my partner.

Why is that a problem?
I become snappy with my partner because I am so unhappy with myself.

Why is that a problem?
He becomes snappy in return.

Why is that a problem?
We fight.

Why is that a problem?
We feel angry with each other and it destroys our bond and weakens our relationship.

And so on. Continue finding the links for as long as it takes. You'll know when you're truly done.

The key is to link the pain you usually associate with the outcome to the behaviour that creates the results you've been experiencing. The behaviour is the only thing you can actually influence, and it's usually also the root of the original and many other associated problems.

Question two: What has it cost me in the past (physically, emotionally, financially, spiritually, relationship-wise and in every other way) to *indulge in the need to eat damaging junk food*?

This is about linking all the times in the past where this behaviour has cost you and what, specifically, it has cost you. Be as specific and unrelenting as possible in getting it all down on paper. 'What else has it cost me?' 'How else has it cost me?' 'Who else was hurt or even damaged because I engaged in this behaviour?' Remember, link as much pain and suffering as possible to the unhelpful behaviour. Do your worst. This isn't about drumming up your guilt for the long term, but if it's there, use it to your advantage in the context of this exercise now. You can choose to release all of these feelings and emotions later and be grateful for them all. Once this question is answered completely, move on to question three.

Question three: What will it cost me in the future (physically, emotionally, financially, spiritually, relationship-wise and in every other way) to *indulge in the need to eat damaging junk food*?

For me, this part of the exercise is one of the most rewarding. Give yourself the time and write as much as you can drag out of your conscious and subconscious mind. Really focus and give it your best. One of the things that made me stop chocolate altogether and release the hold it had on me was acknowledging the cost of sugar in my beloved grandmother's life. I saw her become paralysed and die a sad death after having a heart attack as a result of uncontrolled blood-sugar levels (she was a diabetic and indulged in sweets from time to time).

That insight finally connected me to the understanding that I was digging my own grave. I was following a similar path. I could link so much of my pain to my behaviour. Suddenly, as I was completing this exercise, change became a *must*. And right then, I was free.

However, this freedom came about because of the stacking I'd done – everything I'd written previously throughout the exercise. Don't just skip to the end of this step. It will not work unless you systematically and methodically go through this process. Write it *all* down and free yourself from whatever addiction had a hold on you when you started the exercise. You'll be so grateful to yourself for making the effort and taking the time. This is one of the exercises I often have people who are participating in any of my fertility programs do; because when done properly, it can be utterly life-changing.

During The Fertility Challenge™, for example, after completing the exercise, people typically send me a video describing their experience. They're usually elated and often surprised by the results. Whenever I watch these videos, I'm reminded that that change in perspective is the ultimate miracle, these are powerful moments for participants and for me. I've shed many a tear of gratitude for being able to serve at ever-growing levels.

When you've wrung out every last cost for question three, wrap it up and move on to question four. But before you do, let's talk emotional leverage for a moment…

• HOW TO CREATE EVEN MORE LEVERAGE, ON DEMAND •

Permanent change happens when you create a high level of personal and emotional leverage over yourself. When change became a must for me, I was feeling at my worst. I was overweight, my skin was full of acne and I was lethargic and dealing with a flu that bordered on pneumonia. Needless to say, I was decidedly not where I wanted to be. I'd just completed the costs exercise and was determined that this time, it had to be *very* different (because, of course, I'd promised myself that I would quit chocolate in the past and it hadn't worked). Something radical was required.

I'd read an article about weight loss through the power of the mind. I didn't really connect with the information, but I got one idea that changed everything. It was based on a neuro-linguistic programming technique of replacing the thing you love the most with something utterly disgusting in your mind. I did this every time I thought of chocolate. But I took it to a whole other level. I decided that if, for the next year, I brought any kind of chocolate to my mouth, it would have to be with an equal amount of my own poo. Every time I thought of chocolate, the abominable image of me eating my own poo immediately followed. It nearly made me want to puke – because I was 100% ready to follow through; there was no letting myself off the hook this time. What I found was that because I was fully committed to this crazy idea and fully prepared to follow through, I never had to. (So don't let yourself off the hook.)

Unexpectedly, what happened in a short period of time was that the mere thought of chocolate left the building; it became too disgusting for recollection. When the year was up, there was no way in the universe I was going to touch the stuff any time soon. Literally, the idea of it had become that disgusting. Only five years later was I curious about what would happen if I ate chocolate again. The infatuation was decidedly broken, and thousands of my patients have benefited from my commitment to the cause. Now, as your prize for making it this far into the book, you can too.

Question four: What will I gain and how will I benefit in my life (physically, emotionally, financially, spiritually, relationship-wise and in every other way) by choosing to *let go of the need to indulge in damaging junk food*?

Be sure to write as many possible gains and benefits as your creative brain can dream up. Do your best. Done properly, this exercise is a marvellous, foundational catapult to life-changing results.

I like to keep these lists handy when I'm done, and I recommend you do the same. Consistently review them to keep yourself moving in the direction you envision. Once you've broken the infatuation with the old behaviour and can see that your life can and will be so much better off without it, it's time to implement the next step for your highest good and that of all concerned.

Step 3 – Flow with it

In nature, nothing is static. The macrocosms and microcosms of which we're a part are in constant flow. But when we give in to fear, we crave certainty and security, and we tend to make everything about us and how much we're suffering. This view of the world further strengthens this vicious cycle, which begets contraction and rigidity (in feeling and thinking). This seemingly permanent condition is the opposite of the desired states of being that make us feel relaxed and grateful for our lives, despite things not always being exactly how we'd like them.

Mindfulness helps us experience the difference between 'I *have to* eat well and avoid junk food' and 'I *get to* eat well and avoid junk food'. The former is an inconvenient obligation, the latter a prayer of gratitude. Mindfulness is an incredibly effective tool to help people deal with the stressors of daily life, mood instabilities and the grief of infertility, miscarriage and stillbirth.[33,34,35] Typically, difficult feelings left unacknowledged lead people to a higher likelihood of overeating and making poor choices regarding food.[36,37] They also create or exacerbate many other avoidable health concerns.[38,39] Conversely, a regular mindfulness practice delivers multiple health and fertility benefits, including improvement of erectile dysfunction,[40] hormonal balance (metabolic, stress and reproductive hormones),[41,42] increased conception chances and the ability to take a healthy pregnancy to term.[43,44,45,46]

In the past, whenever I mentioned meditation (another highly effective mindfulness tool) to my patients, their eyes glazed over, and objections regarding lack of time and difficulty 'getting it right' abounded. So, I kept on searching and eventually came across the ancient Buddhist teaching and mindfulness tool called RAIN (which is now scientifically validated).[47,48,49,50,51,52,53,54,55]

RAIN is an acronym that stands for recognise, accept, inquire and note (or non-identify). What I love about RAIN is that it's quick to use and easy to apply. And the more you exercise it, the more it helps you transmute daily challenges and gain many associated health benefits.

'Recognise' is about pausing to acknowledge and connect with the fact that you're feeling stuck. There's no need for any label, story or self-judgement – just recognition of what is. For example, if you're experiencing a craving of some kind, you connect with that fact. Recognising is about being consciously aware that something is present and that it feels a certain way. It's that simple.

Then we 'accept'. It's that moment where, instead of trying to run and/or fight what is, we mentally and energetically lean in to the discomfort and allow it. We embrace and accept it for what it is. So, if you're having a craving, experience and fully open yourself up to the texture of the feeling or the emotion it elicits. Remember, what we resist persists. Just allow what is, without the need to judge it or make it any different. Instead of trying to subdue or eradicate the discomfort of abstaining, give yourself to the perception of that feeling. Sense it and experience it fully. There's no point trying to hide the elephant in the room. Simply appreciate its grace and presence. The *R* and *A* in RAIN allow you to fully implement the first step in the Life Changer Method™ – they allow you to *face it*. Whatever *it* is. Without judgement. So you can apply curious inquiry to what's in front of you and *feel it*.

Once acceptance is in place, the next step is to 'inquire'. Typically, our immediate reaction to a difficult situation is one of aversion, but when we investigate the cause of our suffering more deeply, it's possible to experience a shift in our perception and reaction and not get stuck in any given situation. I like to ask myself, 'What is this situation/challenge/perceived difficulty trying to teach or show me right now?' Another wonderful question is 'How does this serve me – just as it is?' Because ultimately, everything serves. The key is to allow this possibility (rather than to reject it), so you can discover how.

Apply natural curiosity to uncover the layers that momentarily cloud your understanding. Once we make meaning out of our challenges, they transform before our hearts and eyes. Here are some great questions to get you started on your self-exploration with curiosity: 'Where does this feeling want to lead me?' 'What am I perceiving is missing right now?' 'What am I really craving?' 'What if there was nothing missing and everything I need is already within me, right now?' 'What do I need to give or show myself?' 'How do

I need to nurture myself right now?' You'll no doubt come up with more great questions of your own as you lean in to this process.

Finally, the *N* (note or non-identify) in the practice of RAIN allows for what mindfulness teacher Tara Brach describes as a 'natural loving awareness' of the entire situation.[56] Here, you observe and *flow with* the situation. You don't try to fight it or rationalise it. It's almost as if you're a third-party observer – without any attachment, whatsoever, to the outcome. This enables you to see that you are not your 'problem' and, in fact, you have no problems. From this vantage point, a 'problem' can be defined as a single-sided perception of an otherwise (in the greater scheme of things) perfect situation. The gains from any perceived challenge are proportional to the effort required to conquer it. This is no philosophical meandering – this is a practical, physical law of nature. In nature, there is no positive without a negative and vice versa, even when we wish it weren't so.[57]

Whatever the situation, it exists outside of you. You don't own it or belong to it. The true *you* isn't fused or bound (unless you choose to be) to any self-limiting belief, emotion, sensation or story the small self may have once got hooked on. The *N* requires no action. You simply, candidly and compassionately, observe. And the more you do, the more you understand who you are, what you are and how you serve. In turn, you understand how everything and everyone serves you (cravings, difficulties and challenges included). In essence, rather than choosing to be rigidly attached to any one thing or point of view, you *flow with it.*

A parting note on the Life Changer Method™

This isn't a process you'll go through once. It's not like being cured of some rare ailment. It's like bathing. For your sake (as well as the sake of those around you), I hope that you engage in both bathing and the Life Changer Method™ regularly. Practice and conditioning (revising your answer lists and reconnecting with what you have learned throughout the implementation of each step in this process) are vital when it comes to making lasting change.

I recommend you review the lists you made in Step 2 at least once a week for the first three months post completing this exercise, and then at least monthly for a year (adding to your answers each time, if necessary and new things come to mind). As for Steps 1 and 3, let them be your constant, helpful companions.

Each of us is a project, a work of art, a labour of constant conditioning and never-ending improvement. The sooner you accept this, the sooner you can advance in your daily practice of the Life Changer Method™ and know you exist in an ever-evolving and expanding cycle. The moment we have a handle on something at the outermost edge of our comfort zone is the moment that bubble expands to incorporate new opportunities and challenges that keep us growing.

The choice is always yours. You can choose to be willingly in the flow of life (sometimes gentle, sometimes fast and sometimes furious), always moving and growing with the help of tools such as the Life Changer Method™. Or, you can choose to stagnate and let external circumstances govern your reactions. You can stay in your unwillingness and feel as if you're being dragged through deep pain and heartache. But decide you must. Will you learn through love or through pain? I certainly know which I prefer.

You're free to choose what feels best for you. I recommend that you use and reuse this tool to your greatest advantage in every area of your life. Go ahead and use it with everything. The worst thing that will happen is that you'll learn something you can put to good use at some point down the track.

And when it comes to engaging in the practice of optimising your health and fertility, you could have no better ally or greater cheerleader than me in your corner. I know you can do this. Now prove it to yourself.

MIRACLE MOMENTS

• WE WERE WINGING IT •
MEGAN AND JOSH

We felt like any normal young couple doing the usual things. We'd get married, have kids, build a life together, go through the normal progression. But that's not what happened for us. When we lost our first baby to an ectopic pregnancy, we consoled ourselves with the thought that at least we could get pregnant – we looked on the bright side of a dim situation. But when we lost our second baby to miscarriage, we really started to lose hope. There was nothing bright. We both became depressed.

We carried on hoping to get pregnant, doing the same normal things. Of course, we were winging it. We made no lifestyle changes, we bought over-the-counter supplements from the chemist. We didn't change our diets. Until we met Gabriela.

After doing an extensive assessment, Gabriela gave us a list of tasks to do, and an action plan. She helped us address all the minor factors – many things we'd never even considered were stopping us. In our case there were thyroid issues, sperm abnormalities and every little thing that made us not feel and be our best.

Gabriela's approach was far from just talk. It was all about action. She didn't want us to chat about what we needed to do. She expected us to change, for our greater good.

With Gabriela's help, we took some time to look after each other, mourn our loss and really get started on taking the actions she prescribed. With the support of my husband we followed Gabriela's guidelines together. It was challenging adjusting our lifestyle, but we gained so much insight about what we were consuming and the technology and chemicals that harmed us – and as a result, our general health improved dramatically!

It was a long road before we finally conceived, but it was well worth it, especially knowing we would be giving our baby the healthiest start. We thought we might be pregnant and went for an ultrasound. It was astounding – there wasn't one but three hearts beating. We had conceived three babies naturally.

It was a high-risk pregnancy, but we were in great shape, and went on to deliver three beautiful baby boys. It was incredible. But that's not where our story ends. After the boys, we revisited everything we'd learned the first time around and we again very easily and quickly conceived, and carried another healthy (single this time, thankfully!) pregnancy to term and gave birth to an adorable little girl. Our family is now complete. Thank you, Gabriela! I give so much credit to Gabriela for the path she has led us on and to *us*, too, for persevering, making changes, remaining strong and having a little faith.

Fertility Reset Prescription 4: Choose flow

Now it's your turn to apply the Life Changer Method™ to any aspect of your life you'd like to improve upon. Go right ahead, and when you're done, give yourself a high five and go for a massage or a walk or do any other self-nurturing activity you enjoy that will help you keep up the momentum you've created for yourself.

Resources

In the interactive book portal, I've included a whole month's worth of delicious, fertility-boosting meal plans and recipe ideas to help you and your partner nourish your bodies towards creating your ultimate outcome. I've also included some other resources on how to apply the Life Changer Method™. Finally, have you ever wondered how excess weight can impact your fertility? Learn more about this and get your extra goodies at http://thefertile.me/BreakthroughBook.

References

1   Chiu, Y.-H., et al., Association between pesticide residue intake from consumption of fruits and vegetables and pregnancy outcomes among women undergoing infertility treatment with assisted reproductive technology. *JAMA Internal Medicine*, 2018. 178(1).

2   Di Nisio, A., et al., Water and soil pollution as determinant of water and food quality/contamination and its impact on male fertility. *Reproductive Biology and Endocrinology: RB&E*, 2019. 17(1).

3   Barański, M., et al., Higher antioxidant and lower cadmium concentrations and lower incidence of pesticide residues in organically grown crops: A systematic literature review and meta-analyses. *The British Journal of Nutrition*, 2014. 112(5).

4   Dai, Z., et al., Amino acid metabolism in intestinal bacteria and its potential implications for mammalian reproduction. *Molecular Human Reproduction*, 2015. 21(5).

5   Hemmings, K.E., et al., Amino acid turnover by human oocytes is influenced by gamete developmental competence, patient characteristics and gonadotrophin treatment. *Human Reproduction* (Oxford, England), 2013. 28(4).

6   Hibbeln, J.R., et al., Meat meat consumption during pregnancy and substance misuse among adolescent offspring: Stratification of TCN2 genetic variants. *Alcoholism, Clinical and Experimental Research*, 2017. 41(11).

7   Mumford, S.L., et al., Dietary fat intake and reproductive hormone concentrations and ovulation in regularly menstruating women. *The American Journal of Clinical Nutrition*, 2016. 103(3).

8 Nassan, F.L., et al., Intake of protein-rich foods in relation to outcomes of infertility treatment with assisted reproductive technologies. *The American Journal of Clinical Nutrition*, 2018. 108(5).

9 Rink, S.M., et al., Self-report of fruit and vegetable intake that meets the 5 a day recommendation is associated with reduced levels of oxidative stress biomarkers and increased levels of antioxidant defense in premenopausal women. *Journal of the Academy of Nutrition and Dietetics*, 2013. 113(6).

10 Salas-Huetos, A., et al., Dietary patterns, foods and nutrients in male fertility parameters and fecundability: A systematic review of observational studies. *Human Reproduction Update*, 2017. 23(4).

11 Średnicka-Tober, D., et al., Composition differences between organic and conventional meat: A systematic literature review and meta-analysis. *The British Journal of Nutrition*, 2016. 115(6).

12 Sun, Y., et al., Inverse association between organic food purchase and diabetes mellitus in US adults. *Nutrients*, 2018. 10(12).

13 Xia, W., et al., Men's meat intake and treatment outcomes among couples undergoing assisted reproduction. *Fertility and Sterility*, 2015. 104(4).

14 Berthoud, H.-R., et al., Blaming the brain for obesity: Integration of hedonic and homeostatic mechanisms. *Gastroenterology*, 2017. 152(7).

15 Lee, P.C., et al., Food for thought: Reward mechanisms and hedonic overeating in obesity. *Current Obesity Reports*, 2017. 6(4).

16 Arab, A., et al., Dietary patterns and semen quality: A systematic review and meta-analysis of observational studies. *Andrology*, 2018. 6(1).

17 Chavarro, J.E., et al., Iron intake and risk of ovulatory infertility. *Obstetrics and Gynecology*, 2006. 108(5).

18 Liu, C.-Y., et al., The association between dietary patterns and semen quality in a general Asian population of 7282 males. *PLoS One*, 2015. 10(7).

19 Twigt, J.M., et al., The preconception diet is associated with the chance of ongoing pregnancy in women undergoing IVF/ICSI treatment. *Human Reproduction* (Oxford, England), 2012. 27(8).

20 Chen, F., et al., Increased BOLD signals in dlPFC is associated with stronger self-control in food-related decision-making. *Frontiers in Psychiatry*, 2018. 9.

21 Giuliani, N.R., et al., Neural predictors of eating behavior and dietary change. *Annals of the New York Academy of Sciences*, 2018. 1428(1).

22 Werthmann, J., et al., Make up your mind about food: A healthy mindset attenuates attention for high-calorie food in restrained eaters. *Appetite*, 2016. 105.

23 Yokum, S., et al., Cognitive regulation of food craving: Effects of three cognitive reappraisal strategies on neural response to palatable foods. *International Journal of Obesity* (2005), 2013. 37(12).

24 Andre, L., et al., Motivational power of future time perspective: Meta-analyses in education, work, and health. *PLoS One*, 2018. 13(1).

25 Eyal, T., et al., When values matter: Expressing values in behavioral intentions for the near vs. distant future. *Journal of Experimental Social Psychology*, 2009. 45(1).

26 Keller, G., *The ONE Thing: The Surprisingly Simple Truth Behind Extraordinary Results.* 2013: Bard Press.

27 Robbins, T., *Awaken the Giant Within: How to Take Immediate Control of Your Mental, Emotional, Physical and Financial Destiny!* 1992: Free Press.

28 Esterling, B.A., et al., Empirical foundations for writing in prevention and psychotherapy: Mental and physical health outcomes. *Clinical Psychology Review*, 1999. 19(1).

29 Gortner, E.-M., et al., Benefits of expressive writing in lowering rumination and depressive symptoms. *Behavior Therapy*, 2006. 37(3).

30 Hagger, M.S., et al., Interpersonal style should be included in taxonomies of behavior change techniques. *Frontiers in Psychology*, 2014. 5.

31 Hardcastle, S.J., et al., Motivating the unmotivated: How can health behavior be changed in those unwilling to change? *Frontiers in Psychology*, 2015. 6.

32 Hardcastle, S.J., et al., Effectiveness of a motivational interviewing intervention on weight loss, physical activity and cardiovascular disease risk factors: A randomised controlled trial with a 12-month post-intervention follow-up. *The International Journal of Behavioral Nutrition and Physical Activity*, 2013. 10.

33 Huberty, J., et al., Relationship between mindfulness and posttraumatic stress in women who experienced stillbirth. *Journal of Obstetric, Gynecologic, and Neonatal Nursing: JOGNN*, 2018. 47(6).

34 Khoury, B., et al., Mindfulness-based stress reduction for healthy individuals: A meta-analysis. *Journal of Psychosomatic Research*, 2015. 78(6).

35 Nery, S.F., et al., Mindfulness-based program for stress reduction in infertile women: Randomized controlled trial. *Stress and Health: Journal of the International Society for the Investigation of Stress*, 2018.

36 Devonport, T.J., et al., A systematic review of the association between emotions and eating behaviour in normal and overweight adult populations. *Journal of Health Psychology*, 2017.

37 Evers, C., et al., Feeling bad or feeling good, does emotion affect your consumption of food? A meta-analysis of the experimental evidence. *Neuroscience and Biobehavioral Reviews*, 2018. 92.

38 Fava, G.A., et al., Current psychosomatic practice. *Psychotherapy and Psychosomatics*, 2017. 86(1).

39 Fava, G.A., et al., The clinical domains of psychosomatic medicine. *The Journal of Clinical Psychiatry*, 2005. 66(7).

40 Bossio, J.A., et al., Mindfulness-based group therapy for men with situational erectile dysfunction: A mixed-methods feasibility analysis and pilot study. *The Journal of Sexual Medicine*, 2018. 15(10).

41 Pascoe, M.C., et al., Mindfulness mediates the physiological markers of stress: Systematic review and meta-analysis. *Journal of Psychiatric Research*, 2017. 95.

42 Taren, A.A., et al., Mindfulness meditation training alters stress-related amygdala resting state functional connectivity: A randomized controlled trial. *Social Cognitive and Affective Neuroscience*, 2015. 10(12).

43 Domar, A.D., et al., Impact of a group mind/body intervention on pregnancy rates in IVF patients. *Fertility and Sterility*, 2011. 95(7).

44 Galhardo, A., et al., Mindfulness-based program for infertility: Efficacy study. *Fertility and Sterility*, 2013. 100(4).

45 Li, J., et al., Effects of a mindfulness-based intervention on fertility quality of life and pregnancy rates among women subjected to first in vitro fertilization treatment. *Behaviour Research and Therapy*, 2016. 77.

46 Rooney, K.L., et al., The relationship between stress and infertility. *Dialogues in Clinical Neuroscience*, 2018. 20(1).

47 Brewer, J.A., et al., Why is it so hard to pay attention, or is it? Mindfulness, the factors of awakening and reward-based learning. *Mindfulness*, 2013. 4(1).

48 Brewer, J.A., et al., Craving to quit: Psychological models and neurobiological mechanisms of mindfulness training as treatment for addictions. *Psychology of Addictive Behaviors: Journal of the Society of Psychologists in Addictive Behaviors*, 2013. 27(2).

49 Brewer, J.A., et al., Can mindfulness address maladaptive eating behaviors? Why traditional diet plans fail and how new mechanistic insights may lead to novel interventions. *Frontiers in Psychology*, 2018. 9.

50 Elwafi, H.M., et al., Mindfulness training for smoking cessation: Moderation of the relationship between craving and cigarette use. *Drug and Alcohol Dependence*, 2013. 130(1–3).

51 Fulwiler, C., et al., Mindfulness-based interventions for weight loss and CVD risk management. *Current Cardiovascular Risk Reports*, 2015. 9(10).

52   Garrison, K.A., et al., Craving to quit: A randomized controlled trial of smartphone app-based mindfulness training for smoking cessation. *Nicotine & Tobacco Research: Official Journal of the Society for Research on Nicotine and Tobacco*, 2018.

53   Garrison, K.A., et al., Meditation leads to reduced default mode network activity beyond an active task. *Cognitive, Affective & Behavioral Neuroscience*, 2015. 15(3).

54   Loucks, E.B., et al., Mindfulness and cardiovascular disease risk: State of the evidence, plausible mechanisms, and theoretical framework. *Current Cardiology Reports*, 2015. 17(12).

55   Mason, A.E., et al., Testing a mobile mindful eating intervention targeting craving-related eating: Feasibility and proof of concept. *Journal of Behavioral Medicine*, 2018. 41(2).

56   Brach, T. *True Refuge: Finding Peace and Freedom in Your Own Awakened Heart.* 2013, London, UK: Hay House.

57   Feynman, R., *The Feynman Lectures on Physics: Mainly Electromagnetism and Matter.* Vol. 2. 1977: Addison-Wesley.

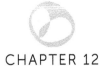

CHAPTER 12

Prescription 5:
Eat Your Way
To Parenthood

'The hardest thing to explain is
the glaringly evident which everybody
had decided not to see.'

Ayn Rand

We have arrived a time in human existence where finally there is now clear and objective consensus in the scientific literature that what we eat not only directly correlates with our fertility but also dictates the health of our offspring and subsequent generations.[1,2,3,4,5,6] If these reasons aren't enough to elicit the desire to do your best in this regard, be sure to complete the Life Changer Method™ outlined under Prescription 4 without delay.

When considering healthy eating, it's important to factor in how food sensitivities and even allergies may affect you, your ability to conceive, your pregnancy and the health of your offspring.[7,8,9,10,11,12]

• FOOD SENSITIVITIES AND ALLERGIES, AND THEIR IMPACT ON YOUR FERTILITY •

Your immune system and your fertility are closely related. In the scientific literature, there's growing evidence of immunological infertility.[13,14,15,16,17,18] Given the fluid nature of our bodily systems, I believe food sensitivity or intolerance can spark a chain of biochemical events which, given certain individual circumstances, can trigger the immune system undesirably, which may even decrease a couple's chances of initially getting pregnant and/or taking a healthy pregnancy to term. I've been a clinician since 2001. I've devoted, conservatively, more than 25,000 hours to the treatment of thousands of patients, and I continue to keenly observe and amass strong empirical data which evidences the dramatic impact dietary modification exerts on a couple's fertility. This, in conjunction with my research, leads me to conclude that in the case of couples experiencing difficulty conceiving or taking home a healthy baby, a carefully considered diet is necessary – no matter what strategy they're using to achieve conception, but especially when ART (IVF/ICSI) are part of the process.[19,20,21,22]

It's now commonly accepted that approximately 70% to 80% of one's immune system 'lives in the gut'.[23,24] So it makes sense that healthy digestion accounts for a healthy immune system. Consequently, the health of our beneficial microorganisms environment (the microbiome), how our food is processed through the digestive canal and how that entire system functions will also have a bearing on optimum fertility.[25,26,27,28,29]

Can you see how simply injecting yourself with hormones isn't the answer when it comes to optimising your chances of conception and a healthy baby – especially if it hasn't already worked?

It isn't only food sensitivities that inflame the immune system. Conception equally arouses an immune response because the body initially perceives the embryo to be foreign. An 'over-reaction' of the immune system may translate into a defence mounted against the developing embryo. Some researchers believe that increased irritation and inflammation of the gut and the reproductive tract (possibly due to allergies and other aggravating substances), combined with an overactive immune response, may damage the embryo, decrease uterine receptivity for implantation and possibly even lead to miscarriage.[30,31,32] As well, we now know that parents with allergies (particularly allergies triggered around the time of conception) may pass their allergies on to a developing baby.[33,34,35,36,37,38]

Constant immune assault from toxins or allergens may turn the body against itself, leading to increased autoimmunity (with elevated autoimmune antibodies) and, eventually, conditions that negatively affect fertility. Because of the situation my patients already find themselves in, due to subfertility or infertility and recurrent miscarriage, I'm very conservative – in the eyes of some, perhaps severe. I recommend that my patients avoid all known (and even potential) allergens while in the preconception preparation period and as many as possible in pregnancy. But if they have a medically diagnosed food allergy, they must *completely avoid* all allergens during the preparatory stage and throughout the entire pregnancy as well.

My view on this is simple. I believe optimum fertility is derived from a complex biochemical chain reaction that must be fine-tuned and reset – especially when things aren't working as they should or as expected. My view is, why would one knowingly risk a negative outcome?

Unfortunately, food sensitivities are often much more difficult to pick up on than full-blown allergies or intolerances. But no matter how silent they may seem, their impact in the grand scheme of taking home a healthy baby must not be underestimated, especially when everything else has failed.

Table 4.1: Most common food intolerances and sensitivities

Most common food intolerances and sensitivities[39]	Prevalence	
Dairy (including but not only lactose intolerance)	~75%	3 in 4 people
Yeast (eg candida infections)	~33%	1 in 3 people
Gluten (including wheat intolerance and coeliac disease)	~15%	1 in 7 people
Fructose and/or sugar	~35%	1 in 3 people
Miscellaneous foods (including food additives)	~1%	1 in 100 people

To get a proper diagnosis, you must work alongside an experienced team familiar with investigating and diagnosing food sensitivities and intolerances. The first step regarding this type of exploration will always be to adjust your diet (to replace the offending foods) rather than go on the long wild goose chase that food allergy tests can take you on without having done the initial ground work.

In the case of the patients I see, and in my clinical experience, the two worst offenders in our modern diets are gluten and dairy. But you must be careful and aware when making the transition to a healthier diet. Most people, unfortunately, end up replacing these ingredients with equally undesirable ones, such as chemical-laden, pre-packaged 'gluten-free' or 'dairy-free' alternatives – the junk varieties found on the shelves of most supermarkets and health food stores. These will not in the least benefit your fertility and your chances of taking home a healthy baby. You must focus instead on what I'll discuss shortly regarding how best to optimise your nutrition.

Meanwhile, I want to educate you about the negative impact gluten, dairy and trans fats can have on reproductive function. If you make the wrong choices while making this change, you won't get any of the benefits of avoiding these damaging foods.

Let's start with gluten. Gluten is scientifically proven to cause infertility, miscarriage and many other health problems for couples who have an intolerance or sensitivity to this highly allergenic protein.[10,40,41,42] The problem is that often, this minor factor or abnormality (ie a mild sensitivity to gluten) isn't picked up on as part of a standard fertility workup. But it has devastating effects. The easiest way to address this situation, in my opinion, is to replace gluten altogether with healthier alternatives.

Even if you don't think gluten is a problem for you, it's only by avoiding it for a few months and then reintroducing it that you'll truly notice the symptoms. These symptoms will typically be significant (even if you've never noticed them before) precisely because of the highly allergenic nature of the offending substance. Previously, you would have not linked the two. When you've been eating gluten for a while, you become accustomed to these slightly bothersome symptoms, often dismissing them as 'normal'. But 'slightly bothersome' on the surface can mean truly devastating for that biochemical chain reaction we want to optimise. Hence the importance of taking this step seriously and wiping the proverbial slate clean. My patients' babies continue to prove to me that this step is a critically important part of a solid strategy. The details of what you need to look out for and what you must do to achieve the best possible results are described in my book *Eat Your Way to Parenthood: The Diet Secrets of Highly Fertile Couples Revealed*.

MIRACLE MOMENTS

• STOP DRINKING THE 'GOGO JUICE' •
TRACEY AND PAUL

We had waited (too) patiently for a decade to get pregnant before finally, I (Tracey) started panicking that I might be getting too old.

I bought into the mumbo jumbo sold at our local chemist, and then a trip to my doctor resulted in a cursory and unsatisfactory 'Here's the referral for your local IVF clinic. See you later.'

The IVF emotional rollercoaster didn't bring success, even though we faithfully did everything required to get pregnant. We undertook two rounds of treatment.

Luckily, we were introduced to Gabriela, and a shift happened. We joined the program, we became committed, we switched gears.

I junked the gym 'gogo juices' in favour of the whole lemon drink, and I dropped weight and was feeling great. I started taking my customised herbs and supplements prescription, that continued to be fine-tuned throughout our treatment especially for me after all my investigations with Gabriela and her team were completed, and got rid of a number of irritating medical issues at the same time. Paul lost weight too. We went on a six-week trip to the USA with our new positive mindset, our approved lifestyle plan and a bag full of supplements. I finally felt attuned to my body; I could almost feel the eggs dropping.

> When Gabriela said we could start trying to conceive, I became pregnant on the first month of trying, a testament to what the body is capable of if you give it the right nourishment and environment. We have a renewed sense of fulfilment, happiness and a beautiful boy, Tyler. We're so grateful to Gabriela and her structured program.

As I briefly discussed, there's one major problem when implementing a gluten-free diet: people often think that everything that says 'gluten-free' on the label is good to eat. Perish that thought. Avoid commercially available gluten-free products with the same focus and intensity as you avoid commercially available gluten-containing varieties. Many of the 'gluten-free' products include nasty ingredients such as soy, trans fats and many other food additives, including health-damaging preservatives. All these food additives must be avoided if you want to optimise your fertility. The best replacements are the least-processed foods (such as vegetables, proteins and good fats), so this new way of nourishing your body does require some advance planning and organisation. But this is a small price to pay for your optimum health and fertility.

Next let's talk about dairy. Although calcium is an essential nutrient for strong bones and optimum sperm and egg quality, dairy isn't the only option when it comes to getting enough calcium. Plus, a good calcium supplement, prescribed by the practitioner treating you, is a great insurance policy.

Table 5.1: Foods rich in calcium

Food	Calcium per 100 g[43]
Sesame seeds	975 mg
Chia seeds	631 mg
Feta (for comparison purposes)	493 mg
Sardines	400 mg
Almonds (raw)	269 mg
Flax seeds	255 mg
Turnip greens (raw)	190 mg
Goji berries (dried)	190 mg
Dandelion leaves (raw)	187 mg
Garlic (raw)	181 mg
Kelp (raw)	168 mg
Figs (dried)	162 mg
Brazil nuts (raw)	160 mg
Kale (cooked)	150 mg
Tahini	143 mg
Collard greens (cooked)	141 mg
Parsley (fresh)	138 mg
Spinach (cooked)	136 mg
Mung beans (raw)	132 mg
Cow's milk (for comparison purposes)	125 mg
Broccoli (cooked)	118 mg
Beet greens (cooked)	114 mg
Hazelnuts (raw)	114 mg
Pistachios (raw)	105 mg
Chicory greens (raw)	100 mg

Dairy is highly inflammatory, allergenic and mucus forming.[44,45,46] And it doesn't just impact the immune system, as previously discussed – it also plays a role in (reproductive and metabolic) hormonal imbalances and triggers genetic predispositions, which may have long-term adverse effects on your health and fertility.[9,47,48,49,50,51,52]

When I recommend you avoid dairy as much as possible, it applies irrespective of whether you have a full-blown allergy, an intolerance or otherwise. Even if you think your allergy or intolerance is 'mild', avoiding dairy is part of the proven strategy to overcome infertility and miscarriage that I've successfully applied to thousands of my patients over the years. You have everything to gain by implementing it, but of course, the choice is yours.

If you *don't* have a full-blown allergy or severe sensitivity, it's OK to have some gluten and/or dairy a couple of times per month, as your '10% for the soul' indulgence. I highly recommend sticking to this kind of interval for best results throughout your preconception preparation and conception-attempt stages. And yes, this information applies to your partner as well. Not only because fertility is a team sport, but also because male reproductive function and optimum fertility are equally negatively affected by the concerns discussed in this section.[53,54,55,56,57,58]

Now let's talk about the number one fertility killer that experts around the world agree is decimating your chances of getting pregnant and carrying a healthy pregnancy to term.[59,60,61] This major fertility threat is found in seemingly inoffensive places, such as some so-called health foods, and in all types of fried foods, pies, pastries, biscuits, ice creams, cakes and more. The perpetrator? Trans fats. These fats are uncommonly found in nature, but they're easily artificially manufactured when vegetable oils become heated and/or are hydrogenated.

• THE #1 FERTILITY KILLER: TRANS FATS •

Trans fat is a result of the hydrogenation of vegetable oil. Hydrogenation makes fats solid at room temperature. Hydrogenated oils add texture to processed foods and increase the shelf life of packaged products. They're also often reused in deep fryers, as they don't appear to spoil easily. Trans fats are not commonly found in nature, except in trivial amounts in some meat and dairy products.

This unnatural or damaged fat is found in food products you may be consuming on a day-to-day basis, such as (to name but a few):

1. Baked goods (cakes, cookies, pie crusts, crackers containing shortening)

2. Ready-made frostings

3. Most packaged snacks

4. Fried foods (and even 'baked not fried' foods), including potato, corn, and tortilla chips, French fries, donuts and fried chicken

5. Prepared doughs, pizza crusts, canned meals, biscuits, cinnamon rolls, margarine and non-dairy creamers

Even though some of these snack foods might not be fried, trans fats may still be added to enhance cooking times and/or flavour (eg microwave popcorn). These damaged fats must be avoided if you want to optimise your and your partner's fertility.

Also be careful when purchasing packaged (or processed/ fast) 'foods' because even when a product claims to contain 'no trans fats', damaged fats are usually hidden under different names, such as hydrogenated and partially hydrogenated oils. Any product that includes vegetable oils which are cooked or processed generally contains damaged fats; even if not classified as trans fats, they're still going to negatively impact your hormones and cellular building blocks and ultimately your health and fertility.[62,63,64,65,66,67]

Trans fats have been linked to cancer, heart disease and infertility. In one study, it was concluded that every 2% increase in the consumption of energy from trans fats (which, incidentally, is about as much as is present in a small packet of chips) increased the risk of infertility due to ovulation problems by 73%.[61] If that isn't enough reason to eliminate these damaged fats from your diet, researchers have also been able to link trans-fat consumption to male infertility[59,60] and prostate cancer[68,69] as well as sperm and egg quality issues.[59,64,67,70]

The reality is that if you're eating these foods, you're dramatically decreasing your chances of taking home a healthy baby. If you're struggling with replacing these foods with healthier alternatives, go back to Prescription 4 and implement the Life Changer Method™. My patients regularly (gratefully) attest to the effectiveness of this valuable tool, here at your disposal.

Real food is best for your optimum fertility

Meet your new nutritional compass for optimum health and fertility. A simple way to ensure the food you're consuming is real nourishment is to consume only foods that are closest to their natural state (field/farm) as possible. Put simply, you want to eat food you can easily recognise when it's on your plate.

To optimise your fertility, base your meals on vegetables and proteins that have gone through one or two, maximum three, steps from field to plate. Following this strategy, you'll never again need to ask, 'What should I eat?' Eat food that, when it's on your plate, has been changed very little from its natural state (ie when it's growing in the field or being raised on a farm).

Let's use corn (organic, non-GMO of course!) in four different ways as a visual example of what I mean.

1. Corn *on* the cob

2. Corn *off* the cob

3. Popcorn

4. Tortilla chips

Corn is grown in the field as a crop. After being harvested, it's transported to the stores, where you buy it as corn on the cob. You cook it and eat it (ideally with some protein and at least four other vegetables, for a balanced meal). This is one step from field to plate. You've made only one change to the food – cooking it.

Corn off the cob, is similar, except now you've cut the kernels off the cob and likely mixed it into a dish (a salad, for example). This is two steps from field to plate because you added an extra processing step.

Next, you have popcorn – the air-popped variety, not any 'funfair food experiment', which Dr Pam Peeke, author of *The Hunger Fix*,[71] refers to as a poor excuse for food found on most supermarket shelves, such as those packets full of chemicals with corn kernels inside that you're supposed to put in the **gasp** microwave. (Stay. Away. From. All. Of. Those. Including the microwave.) Air-popped corn is three steps from field to plate: corn is grown and harvested, kernels are dehydrated and packaged, and then you cook (pop) them at home.

Finally, we have tortilla chips. These are 'funfair food experiments', which don't lead you to optimum health or fertility. Here's how it works: 1) corn is grown and harvested; 2) kernels are removed from the cob and processed into a pulp; 3) a %@#$ storm of chemicals are added – colourings, flavourings, preservatives and food additives of all kinds; 4) this mixture is shaped, dehydrated, fried and/or whatever else; 5) you get the final product out of a packet full of marketing that tries to convince you how healthy it is with claims such as 'baked not fried' and that it's all going to be OK – when deep down, we know full well it can't be.

Have you ever noticed how nobody tries to tell you on a stalk of broccoli, cabbage or Brussels sprouts how good that stuff is for you? No writing is required, and the best versions (even for the healthy foods) are those that don't even come in packaging. Something to think about.

Therefore, I also recommend to my patients, beyond replacing foods that contain gluten, dairy and trans fats, that all the food they consume be as close to its natural state as possible (maximum three steps from field to plate; ideally one or two). This will go a long way to ensuring that the food you're consuming is real nourishment that your body can use to fuel and renew itself, as well as to optimise your chances of taking home a healthy baby.

Fertility Reset Prescription 5: Out with the old, in with the new

This is a two-step task.

First, you'll create your own meal plan based on the new style of eating I've outlined in this section of the book. You can also visit the interactive book portal to download one of the free sample meal plans for inspiration, along with a blank planner – this will be as simple as choosing your meals according to your eating preferences and slotting them into your plan. If you're creating your own, choose balanced, vital, healthy foods and snacks based on proteins and low-glycaemic vegetables (eg leafy greens and other non-starchy types). Then get your shopping list ready.

Second, pull everything out of your pantry, fridge and freezer. Put it all on the bench or dining table. Figure out which items will get you closer to your dream of having a baby and which won't. Decide what needs to be binned or donated to where it may be appreciated. Now you're ready for your weekly grocery shop. Be sure to stick to your shopping list. Your fertility and prospective child are counting on it.

If this task feels difficult, be sure to implement Prescription 4 as soon as possible.

Resources

As a bonus gift, I've added my book *Eat Your Way to Parenthood: The Diet Secrets of Highly Fertile Couples Revealed* to the interactive portal for this book, in addition to meal plans, shopping lists and your blank planner. Visit http://thefertile.me/BreakthroughBook for everything you need to implement this prescription on your journey to parenthood.

References

1 Day, J., et al., Influence of paternal preconception exposures on their offspring: Through epigenetics to phenotype. *American Journal of Stem Cells*, 2016. 5(1).

2 Kanherkar, R.R., et al., Epigenetics across the human lifespan. *Frontiers in Cell and Developmental Biology*, 2014. 2.

3 Lee, H.-S., Impact of maternal diet on the epigenome during in utero life and the developmental programming of diseases in childhood and adulthood. *Nutrients*, 2015. 7(11).

4   Lorite Mingot, D., et al., Epigenetic effects of the pregnancy
    Mediterranean diet adherence on the offspring metabolic syndrome
    markers. *Journal of Physiology and Biochemistry*, 2017. 73(4).

5   Ornellas, F., et al., Obese fathers lead to an altered metabolism and
    obesity in their children in adulthood: Review of experimental and human
    studies. *Jornal De Pediatria*, 2017. 93(6).

6   Skinner, M.K., et al., Environmentally induced epigenetic
    transgenerational inheritance of sperm epimutations promote genetic
    mutations. *Epigenetics*, 2015. 10(8).

7   Antvorskov, J.C., et al., Association between maternal gluten intake
    and type 1 diabetes in offspring: National prospective cohort study in
    Denmark. *BMJ (Clinical research ed.)*, 2018. 362.

8   Barmeyer, C., et al., Long-term response to gluten-free diet as evidence
    for non-celiac wheat sensitivity in one third of patients with diarrhea-
    dominant and mixed-type irritable bowel syndrome. *International Journal
    of Colorectal Disease*, 2017. 32(1).

9   Kim, K., et al., Dairy food intake is associated with reproductive
    hormones and sporadic anovulation among healthy premenopausal
    women. *The Journal of Nutrition*, 2017. 147(2).

10 Lasa, J.S., et al., Risk of infertility in patients with celiac disease:
    A meta-analysis of observational studies. *Arquivos De Gastroenterologia*,
    2014. 51(2).

11 Venter, C., et al., Maternal dietary intake in pregnancy and lactation and
    allergic disease outcomes in offspring. *Pediatric Allergy and Immunology:
    Official Publication of the European Society of Pediatric Allergy and
    Immunology*, 2017. 28(2).

12 Zhu, Y., et al., Maternal dietary intakes of refined grains during
    pregnancy and growth through the first 7 y of life among children born
    to women with gestational diabetes. *The American Journal of Clinical
    Nutrition*, 2017. 106(1).

13 Brazdova, A., et al., Immune aspects of female infertility.
    International Journal of Fertility & Sterility, 2016. 10(1).

14 Brew, O., et al., The links between maternal histamine levels and
    complications of human pregnancy. *Journal of Reproductive Immunology*,
    2006. 72(1–2).

15 Gray, L.E.K., et al., The maternal diet, gut bacteria, and bacterial
    metabolites during pregnancy influence offspring asthma. *Frontiers in
    Immunology*, 2017. 8.

16 McAllister, B.P., et al., A comprehensive review of celiac disease/gluten-
    sensitive enteropathies. *Clinical Reviews in Allergy & Immunology*, 2018.

17 Patel, B.Y., et al., Food allergy: Common causes, diagnosis, and treatment. *Mayo Clinic Proceedings*, 2015. 90(10).

18 Pinzer, T.C., et al., Circadian profiling reveals higher histamine plasma levels and lower diamine oxidase serum activities in 24% of patients with suspected histamine intolerance compared to food allergy and controls. *Allergy*, 2018. 73(4).

19 Karayiannis, D., et al., Adherence to the Mediterranean diet and IVF success rate among non-obese women attempting fertility. *Human Reproduction* (Oxford, England), 2018. 33(3).

20 Sauder, K.A., et al., Predictors of infant body composition at 5 months of age: The Healthy Start study. *The Journal of Pediatrics*, 2017. 183.

21 Tahir, M.J., et al., Higher maternal diet quality during pregnancy and lactation is associated with lower infant weight-for-length, body fat percent, and fat mass in early postnatal life. *Nutrients*, 2019. 11(3).

22 Vujkovic, M., et al., Associations between dietary patterns and semen quality in men undergoing IVF/ICSI treatment. *Human Reproduction* (Oxford, England), 2009. 24(6).

23 Abdel-Haq, R., et al., Microbiome-microglia connections via the gut-brain axis. *The Journal of Experimental Medicine*, 2019. 216(1).

24 Vighi, G., et al., Allergy and the gastrointestinal system. *Clinical and Experimental Immunology*, 2008. 153(Suppl 1).

25 Aatsinki, A.-K., et al., Gut microbiota composition in mid-pregnancy is associated with gestational weight gain but not prepregnancy body mass index. *Journal of Women's Health* (2002), 2018. 27(10).

26 Chen, C., et al., The microbiota continuum along the female reproductive tract and its relation to uterine-related diseases. *Nature Communications*, 2017. 8.

27 Prince, A.L., et al., The perinatal microbiome and pregnancy: Moving beyond the vaginal microbiome. *Cold Spring Harbor Perspectives in Medicine*, 2015. 5(6).

28 Staude, B., et al., The microbiome and preterm birth: A change in paradigm with profound implications for pathophysiologic concepts and novel therapeutic strategies. *BioMed Research International*, 2018.

29 Tersigni, C., et al., Recurrent pregnancy loss is associated to leaky gut: A novel pathogenic model of endometrium inflammation? *Journal of Translational Medicine*, 2018. 16.

30 Prentice, S., They are are what you eat: Can nutritional factors during gestation and early infancy modulate the neonatal immune response? *Frontiers in Immunology*, 2017. 8.

31 Sirota, I., et al., Potential potential influence of the microbiome on infertility and assisted reproductive technology. *Seminars in Reproductive Medicine*, 2014. 32(1).

32 Sohn, K., et al., Prenatal and postnatal administration of prebiotics and probiotics. *Seminars in Fetal & Neonatal Medicine*, 2017. 22(5).

33 Arshad, S.H., et al., The effect of parental allergy on childhood allergic diseases depends on the sex of the child. *The Journal of Allergy and Clinical Immunology*, 2012. 130(2).

34 Cook-Mills, J.M., Maternal influences over offspring allergic responses. *Current Allergy and Asthma Reports*, 2015. 15(2).

35 Meng, S.-S., et al., Maternal allergic disease history affects childhood allergy development through impairment of neonatal regulatory T-cells. *Respiratory Research*, 2016. 17(1).

36 Mørkve Knudsen, T., et al., Transgenerational and intergenerational epigenetic inheritance in allergic diseases. *The Journal of Allergy and Clinical Immunology*, 2018. 142(3).

37 Svanes, C., et al., Father's environment before conception and asthma risk in his children: A multi-generation analysis of the Respiratory Health In Northern Europe study. *International Journal of Epidemiology*, 2017. 46(1).

38 Tan, L., et al., Neonatal immune state is influenced by maternal allergic rhinitis and associated with regulatory T cells. *Allergy, Asthma & Immunology Research*, 2017. 9(2).

39 Food Intolerance Institute. 2018. Food Sensitivities.

40 Bold, J., et al., Non-coeliac gluten sensitivity and reproductive disorders. *Gastroenterology and Hepatology From Bed to Bench*, 2015. 8(4).

41 Casella, G., et al., Celiac disease and obstetrical-gynecological contribution. *Gastroenterology and Hepatology From Bed to Bench*, 2016. 9(4).

42 Singh, P., et al., Celiac disease in women with infertility: A meta-analysis. *Journal of Clinical Gastroenterology*, 2016. 50(1).

43 United States Department of Agriculture (USDA). 2018. *Food Composition Databases*.

44 Bartley, J., et al., Does milk increase mucus production? *Medical Hypotheses*, 2010. 74(4).

45 Esmaillzadeh, A., et al., Dairy consumption and circulating levels of inflammatory markers among Iranian women. *Public Health Nutrition*, 2010. 13(09).

46 Jianqin, S., et al., Effects of milk containing only A2 beta casein versus milk containing both A1 and A2 beta casein proteins on gastrointestinal physiology, symptoms of discomfort, and cognitive behavior of people with self-reported intolerance to traditional cows' milk. *Nutrition Journal*, 2015. 15(1).

47 Melnik, B.C., et al., Milk is not just food but most likely a genetic transfection system activating mTORC1 signaling for postnatal growth. *Nutrition Journal*, 2013. 12.

48 Melnik, B.C., et al., Milk consumption during pregnancy increases birth weight, a risk factor for the development of diseases of civilization. *Journal of Translational Medicine*, 2015. 13.

49 Melnik, B.C., et al., Milk's role as an epigenetic regulator in health and disease. *Diseases*, 2017. 5(1).

50 Melnik, B.C., et al., Exosomes of pasteurized milk: Potential pathogens of Western diseases. *Journal of Translational Medicine*, 2019. 17.

51 Rajaeieh, G., et al., The relationship between intake of dairy products and polycystic ovary syndrome in women who referred to Isfahan University of Medical Science clinics in 2013. *International Journal of Preventive Medicine*, 2014. 5(6).

52 Wiley, A.S., Cow milk consumption, insulin-like growth factor-I, and human biology: A life history approach. *American Journal of Human Biology: The Official Journal of the Human Biology Council*, 2012. 24(2).

53 Afeiche, M., et al., Dairy food intake in relation to semen quality and reproductive hormone levels among physically active young men. *Human Reproduction* (Oxford, England), 2013. 28(8).

54 Hanson, H.A., et al., Risk of childhood mortality in family members of men with poor semen quality. *Human Reproduction* (Oxford, England), 2017. 32(1).

55 Harper, L., et al., An exploration into the motivation for gluten avoidance in the absence of coeliac disease. *Gastroenterology and Hepatology from Bed to Bench*, 2018. 11(3).

56 Kumar, N., et al., Trends of male factor infertility, an important cause of infertility: A review of literature. *Journal of Human Reproductive Sciences*, 2015. 8(4).

57 Ozgör, B., et al., Coeliac disease and reproductive disorders. *Scandinavian Journal of Gastroenterology*, 2010. 45(4).

58 Rambhatla, A., et al., The role of estrogen modulators in male hypogonadism and infertility. *Reviews in Urology*, 2016. 18(2).

59 Chavarro, J.E., et al., Trans-fatty acid levels in sperm are associated with sperm concentration among men from an infertility clinic. *Fertility and Sterility*, 2011. 95(5).

60 Chavarro, J.E., et al., Trans fatty acid intake is inversely related to total sperm count in young healthy men. *Human Reproduction* (Oxford, England), 2014. 29(3).

61 Chavarro, J.E., et al., Dietary fatty acid intakes and the risk of ovulatory infertility. *The American Journal of Clinical Nutrition*, 2007. 85(1).

62 Arvizu, M., et al., Male dietary trans fat intake is inversely associated to fertilization rates. *Fertility and Sterility*, 2015. 104(3).

63 Attaman, J.A., et al., Dietary fat and semen quality among men attending a fertility clinic. *Human Reproduction* (Oxford, England), 2012. 27(5).

64 Eskew, A.M., et al., The association between fatty acid index and in vitro fertilization outcomes. *Journal of Assisted Reproduction and Genetics*, 2017. 34(12).

65 Missmer, S.A., et al., A prospective study of dietary fat consumption and endometriosis risk. *Human Reproduction* (Oxford, England), 2010. 25(6).

66 Wanders, A.J., et al., Trans fat intake and its dietary sources in general populations worldwide: A systematic review. *Nutrients*, 2017. 9(8).

67 Wise, L.A., et al., Dietary fat intake and fecundability in 2 preconception cohort studies. *American Journal of Epidemiology*, 2018. 187(1).

68 Chavarro, J.E., et al., A prospective study of trans-fatty acid levels in blood and risk of prostate cancer. *Cancer Epidemiology, Biomarkers & Prevention*, 2008. 17(1).

69 Van Blarigan, E.L., et al., Fat intake after prostate cancer diagnosis and mortality in the Physicians' Health Study. *Cancer Causes & Control: CCC*, 2015. 26(8).

70 Chiu, Y.-H., et al., Diet and female fertility: Doctor, what should I eat? *Fertility and Sterility*, 2018. 110(4).

71 Peeke, P., *The Hunger Fix: The Three-Stage Detox and Recovery Plan for Overeating and Food Addiction*. 2013: Rodale Books.

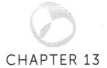

CHAPTER 13

Prescription 6: De-Escalating The Emotional Impact Of Infertility

'Every stumble is not a fall, and every fail does not mean failure.'

Oprah Winfrey

As someone who has experienced infertility first-hand and been a confidant and witness for thousands of people over the last two decades, I've come to understand that our thoughts have immense power. They have the power to uplift us or throw us in the deepest and darkest dungeons of despair.

You get to choose what you focus on at any time.

For instance, when you experience something that displeases you, you have two choices. Choice number one is to see the issue, acknowledge it for what it is and immediately focus on a thought or feeling that makes you happy instead. Choice number two is to engage with the event, the issue, the person, the circumstance you can't change and perpetuate the displeasure.

With choice number two, you give yourself the hedonistic luxury of obsessing about how unjust or unfair things are, and how life never seems to go your way. You may dwell on how much you struggle or have struggled or will continue to struggle because things never change, despite all your hardest and deepest and best efforts. Instead of focusing on what is good, pure and joyful in your life (despite the challenges), your mind turns to what you don't have and how your entire life sucks because of it. This is the perfect breeding ground for wild fantasies that have you imagining that anywhere else would be better than 'here', or that the grass is so much greener for others.

Soon enough, everything becomes coloured by despair. The brain quickly begins to distort, delete and generalise your every experience to match this new standard of how life 'really is'.[1,2] Even if that isn't how life really is. We become incredibly proficient at making ourselves believe whatever we consistently tell ourselves with enough conviction and emotion. Our brains are amazing at finding evidence to prove to ourselves whatever we want to believe – whether it's positive or negative. This type of confirmation bias makes negative thoughts spread in your mind like wildfire.[3]

The emotional challenge posed by infertility is a prime example of how this works. Those who are trying to conceive without the desired result might perceive their situation as 'miserable'. But what if this perception was a choice? You see, without much effort and just enough focus, the untrained brain allows this *pain* to quickly escalate to misery. We choose what meaning we give the pain. The choice is always yours. I know this may feel difficult to accept, and if I hadn't gone through it myself and with my patients, I might even agree with you. But I've seen too much, and I've seen that through self-awareness and steadfast focus, it's possible to live your best life – with or without a baby.

Hold on. Before you burn this book, let me explain. You may think that overcoming fertility struggles and having a baby will make you happy forever more. And that would be nice. But here's what's actually true: if you cannot make yourself feel happy, grateful and alive *right now*, having a baby (or whatever it is you think you want or need to be happy) will not make you feel these things. No matter how much you truly want it or think that it will.

After 25,000 plus hours in clinical practice, talking to patients, treating people from every walk of life (including celebrities), I can tell you that nobody is immune to thinking that something or someone other than ourselves could be responsible for our own happiness. But sooner or later, that myth is debunked, and the truth of a previously false expectation comes to the light.

I promise you this: learning to be happy in your life and within yourself right now, with or without a baby, is the key to being truly happy and enjoying your relationship with your partner. No matter what life throws at you. Now and when you eventually have a baby. Learning to cultivate and nourish your own happiness is the key to becoming the best possible version of yourself and the best parent you can be. It all starts in this moment, from the inside out.

How much longer will you wait? Choose right now to stop being the victim in a life that hasn't yet turned out how you want it to – and take charge. It all begins with you and ends with you. So, if you can't find your strength and work to become the best version of yourself, to be happy with what you already have, right now, you never will.

MIRACLE MOMENTS

• WE GAVE UP TRYING
TO CONTROL THE OUTCOME •
BROOKE AND TOM

Like many other healthy couples in their early thirties, we always assumed that we would get pregnant quickly and easily. So, after six months of trying unsuccessfully, we saw a fertility specialist who couldn't find any specific reason why we weren't getting pregnant (which was great news!). My semen analysis showed mild low morphology but otherwise, I was told, all was normal. Brooke was diagnosed with an underactive thyroid and placed on thyroxine and was also told she had polycystic ovaries (not the syndrome) but that this shouldn't impact getting pregnant. But it did mean that Brooke had an irregular cycle, and it was difficult to pinpoint when she ovulated. So the doctor agreed to monitor the next few cycles while we tried naturally.

But it didn't work, so we moved to the next step – IUI. We hoped that this could overcome my sperm morphology issue and ensure the sperm was actually getting to the eggs. However, after two unsuccessful attempts, we were moved onto IVF. All of a sudden, we were 'that' couple doing ICSI. We put our entire trust into our specialist. We felt like we were on the fast train and couldn't get off. It was moving too quickly.

Like many others, we believed that ICSI was going to be the magic bullet. And our specialist had told us that 80% of couples in our age group were pregnant within two cycles. Unfortunately for us, despite a good number of eggs and embryos reaching blastocyst, we were still not pregnant after two cycles. Now we were one of those couples sitting in the 20% group. By this stage, we felt that the industry was a 'money making machine' and that our specialist didn't care about us or our situation. We were a healthy couple who had spent thousands of dollars and eighteen months trying and failing to get pregnant – yet we still had no answers as to why.

This was when I came across Gabriela. I'd already been on a health kick over the last twelve months, exercising a lot and eating healthy foods, so I was ready to take it to the next level. But Brooke needed a lot of convincing!

We had an initial call with Gabriela, and the assessment we went through was very comprehensive. I was 100% into it but Brooke was still sceptical because she thought 'If ICSI didn't work, how could anything else?' Yet we decided to give it a go. We had nothing to lose.

The biggest positive for Brooke was the in-depth assessment with our primary practitioner in the program. She wanted to know 'why' it hadn't been working. What were the factors stopping us from falling pregnant? We hadn't had this level of analysis with the previous specialist. We were taken back to the drawing board and everything was tested. We discovered many other contributing factors that were interfering with our trying to become parents – factors not considered before.

Brooke's underactive thyroid wasn't well controlled. There was also mild endometriosis. It turned out I had very low semen morphology (not just a mild case, as I'd been previously told), and my sperm's DNA fragmentation, which hadn't been tested before, was very high and impacting our chances. There were also several other small factors that required treatment.

We'd thought we were pretty healthy before the program but realised that the difference between healthy and optimum can be very big – and we now knew how much it was impacting us.

After many months of living healthy, the moment came to actively start trying. Unfortunately, after four months of trying naturally, we were still not pregnant. Those negative feelings crept back in. We'd done all this work on our health and fertility and it didn't work! But it was great to have our practitioner and the team to keep us positive.

We agreed to move back to IVF and to do this in conjunction with the program. This was mainly due to the fact that we'd found out Brooke had a high natural killer cell result and needed immune suppressing drugs to help keep a pregnancy in place.

But this time it was going to be different. We switched doctors (one recommended by Gabriela's clinic), our eggs and semen were top quality (thanks to the program), we would test the embryos before putting them back in – a test known as pre-implantation genetic screening (PGS) – and we would get those natural killer cells under control. And most importantly, we were 100% guided by Gabriela's team throughout the IVF process.

We managed to freeze and bank a number of PGS-tested embryos. However, two transfers still didn't work, even with steroids and intralipids to treat the natural killer cells.

Obviously, this was very upsetting, and at the same time, a personal tragedy happened. It turned out to be one of the most stressful times of our lives. But we weren't going to give up. We wanted it too much. And Gabriela and the team were always by our sides, with such positivity, telling us we would have a baby, it was just a matter of time.

We paused IVF because Brooke was feeling horrible on the steroids and her stress levels at work were incredibly high. We came to the decision that Brooke needed to reduce stress and decided for Brooke to quit her job. The minute she handed in her resignation, she relaxed and started to let go.

On her last day of work, we found out that we were pregnant naturally! After five failed IVF cycles, it was without a doubt the most incredible day of our lives, outside of the day bub was born. We couldn't believe it. We cried in utter surprise, joy, relief and excitement.

We now have the most amazing, healthy little boy who is so, so loved. He is more incredible than we ever imagined, and he was certainly worth the wait.

The pregnancy and birth, and even the first ten weeks of his life, were all made easier by Gabriela's program, as Brooke felt healthy and strong throughout. We are so grateful to have a Gabriela's amazing team around us, we decided to revisit the program to prepare to conceive our second child. After five months of trying naturally, we used one of the frozen embryos stored from our last cycle and couldn't believe it when we were successful straight away. We are thrilled to welcome our second baby boy and we couldn't be happier.

I'm sure I'm not the first person to tell you that what you're experiencing right now doesn't have to stop you from living a joyful, engaging, fulfilling and incredible life. It cannot rob you of having all the love, connection, significance, certainty, fun and growth you want in this lifetime. Unless you choose that it will.

You may need time to think about and deeply consider what I'm saying. You may even need to read and reread this section while asking yourself, 'What if this was true?' (*hint* it is), until you can decide to try the idea on. And that's OK. But if you've made it this far, indulge in this moment a little longer, until at least the end of this section, because right here could lie your breakthrough.

This game (why so serious – what if you turned it into a game?) is about helping you sculpt the best version of yourself. Diamonds are created because of the pressure, not despite of it. A baby doesn't make you into who you need to become, as much as it's a big enough motivator for many people – one worth staying on course for. And what if the possibility of that motivator is the gift of this whole experience for you? What if this whole thing isn't about the baby after all? What if there was a much grander plan in place – for your highest good and the highest good of all concerned? What if this whole thing is all about the contribution you're here to make? We all experience things in life for different reasons, and although it may not be possible, right now, to know why, consider this: what if this is the way life has found to help you become everything you can be in this lifetime?

To borrow from Oprah Winfrey's *What I Know For Sure*, when you conquer your mind, you conquer your life, even against all odds.[4]

Only you can master yourself. And even in this context, mastery is never about the baby. It can help you have the baby, but the gift of mastery remains firmly on the experience and meaning we choose to give the journey. Babies grow up and soon enough flee the nest and then, yet again, you are left with you. Remember, it all begins with you and ends with you. Find your strength and work to become the best version of yourself right now – for yourself. Because it is typically by becoming the person you need to become that you get to experience everything you want in life (not before).

All of this requires a definitive decision backed up by conclusive action. A decision that happens in a heartbeat. The mere fact that you've picked up this book and read this far is all the evidence I need to conclude that it's time for you to take charge and take action. If not now, when? A choice is all it takes. And implementing what you learn throughout this book is where results come from.

• ARE YOU SERIOUS ABOUT THIS? •

Do you really want to change the way infertility and miscarriage make you feel? Then continue reading. Let me show you how.

Your predominant way of perceiving situations and thinking about things becomes your explanatory style, which ultimately becomes the way in which you view and process circumstances in your life. A pessimistic explanatory style is associated with what prominent psychology researcher and author Martin Seligman defined as 'learned helplessness'.[5]

Learned helplessness refers to the belief that failure is inevitable. It is underpinned by three major concepts: permanence, pervasiveness and personalisation.

Permanence relates to the feeling that whatever temporary situation you're currently experiencing will last forever (even if you have plenty of evidence to the contrary – eg other people who experienced miscarriage and/or infertility, in a situation similar to yours, have managed to have a baby). In a moment of 'permanent thinking' there is a feeling that all your worst nightmares will persist indefinitely and there's simply nothing positive that could be drawn from the experience. For instance, 'My ovulation was delayed by three days this month' becomes 'I will never have a baby', or, 'My fertility clinic didn't return my call when they said they would' escalates to 'They clearly can't help me and I'm doomed to be infertile forever'.

Pervasiveness translates to a feeling of generalised, unavoidable catastrophe. For example, 'My partner disagrees with me about an issue' becomes 'Our whole relationship is terrible and doomed to fail', or, 'My partner's fertility results are below average' becomes 'We can never be happy together'.

Personalisation is laced with a veil of guilt that makes everything seem like you're doomed and it's all your fault. For instance, 'If I had done or hadn't done XYZ, I would have a baby by now', or, 'It's all my fault; it's too late'. I'm all for taking charge of my life and teaching my patients to do the same. But it's important to realise there are things simply out of your control – no matter how much you wish the story was different. Even if your previous actions have contributed to an existing situation, you're deserving of your own kindness, love and forgiveness, just as the baby you want to create and any other person is. Embodying this realisation and taking charge of your areas of influence is what can get you closer to your desired result – anything else will just have you spinning and wearing out your wheels.

Holding a grudge and blaming yourself for past instances completely out of your control in the *here and now* is *personalisation*. Persistently describing your circumstances through permanence, pervasiveness and personalisation leads you to learned helplessness and a vicious cycle of anxiety, depression and low self-esteem.[6,7,8,9] In short, it leads you to avoidable suffering. Hanging out in permanence, pervasiveness and/or personalisation for too long doesn't get you closer to the healthy baby of your dreams. And plainly, it makes you miserable before, during and after it is all said and done.

My patients are living proof that through practice, it's possible to replace learned helplessness with learned optimism.[5,10] If you do what I recommend throughout the rest of this section, you will achieve what countless of my patients have been able to create for themselves on their fertility journey: an empowering perspective. You may need additional help, and if that's the case, don't delay seeking professional advice. Your courage and perseverance in working through and choosing to let go of the feelings and emotions that no longer serve you will give you freedom. The new attitude you'll develop will strengthen your resilience and reignite your determination for the work required on your journey to parenthood.

• REWRITE YOUR STORY, BECAUSE ONLY YOU CAN •

This exercise invites you to look at your story, or how you explain aspects of what happens in your life, from a fresh new perspective.

Every time you engage with and practice this new perspective, you move yourself from learned helplessness to learned optimism. In every moment there is only one person who can make this choice, and that is you.

	When something good happens	When something bad happens
Pessimistic explanation	• Temporary • Contained • It involves other people or outside circumstances	• Permanent • Pervasive • Personal
Optimistic explanation	• Permanent • Pervasive • Personal	• Temporary • Contained • It involves other people or outside circumstances

Think of a 'bad' event you have experienced and feel free to write your answers in the space below or a separate sheet of paper:

Now, rewrite the event from a plausible *optimistic* perspective accounting for the fact that whatever happened is temporary and contained and not personal (people do things for their own reasons that have nothing to do with you). In your explanation, remember that (just like the people you love the most in your life) you deserve kindness, forgiveness and love no matter what:

Think of a 'good' event you have experienced:

How would you typically explain it?

Now, rewrite the event from a plausible *optimistic* perspective accounting for the fact that whatever happened is permanent, pervasive and personal:

When learned helplessness becomes ingrained in a person's thinking, pessimistic explanations tend to prevail – hence, the previous prompt for an optimistic explanation. If you tend to be pessimistic, you'll benefit from actively reframing your explanatory style. This exercise is a great way to begin. With it, I'll leave you my gentle reminder that you are blessed, you are breathing and don't *have* to do this – you *get* to do this, now. Isn't that extraordinary? There are millions of people who aren't as fortunate.

'You are not born with a fixed amount of resilience. Like a muscle, you can build it up, draw on it when you need it. In that process you will figure out who you really are – and you just might become the very best version of yourself.'

Sheryl Sandberg

MIRACLE MOMENTS

• LIFE IS FULL OF SURPRISES •
KYLIE AND STEVE

We already had a beautiful daughter, and so we assumed all would be well for our next pregnancy. After trying for two years for our second baby and suffering a miscarriage, we started to worry that we were running out of time and it would never happen.

We thought we had a healthy diet and lifestyle, we exercised, and my cycle was regular. But after the miscarriage, I knew we just couldn't be as healthy as we needed to be. After visiting a fertility specialist, we were disappointed to be told our only solution was IVF.

IVF wasn't a viable option financially, and I had conceived twice previously, so we didn't think it was for me. But I knew that if we did nothing, then five years down the line I'd be devastated and regret not doing everything possible to have a healthy baby. I'm from a large family, the eldest of six.

I knew we couldn't stop at one child. We needed support, guidance and external accountability, because even though I knew what we needed to do, we also needed an extra nudge.

A friend told me about Gabriela and her programs. She'd got pregnant easily after making some of the recommended lifestyle changes. I knew immediately this was the answer we were searching for. So, we joined and began to address the right factors to improve our fertility. We learned about so many things we could do to improve our fertility, and we quickly made the changes required, did the tests we were asked and pretty much implemented everything Gabriela and her team told us to do.

We committed to the program even though we sometimes found it difficult. I lost fifteen kilos easily. Though I didn't enjoy the taste of the supplements and medicines I was prescribed, I just kept my mantra in mind as I took them: 'Baby, baby, baby!'

On our first attempt we got pregnant. I was so surprised, given how long it had taken us to conceive the last time.

But that wasn't even my biggest surprise. Nine months later, while in search of a comfortable position, I didn't realise when I was in established labour and she was crowning. I gave birth, standing upright in the en suite, to our beautiful and healthy baby girl! It was a smooth, easy and fast labour, and she was a dream baby, which I attribute to our improved health as a result of Gabriela's program.

Don't dismiss this message because you think it doesn't apply to you. I promise it applies to you more than it may seem initially – have a 'deep and meaningful' conversation with yourself and be open to discovering the important links and how they apply to your situation.

Allow this message to filter through your heart and your soul so you can incorporate the true meaning of what I'm communicating: *You are already enough. You are already complete. Now. Irrespective of a baby.* No matter what you may have told yourself or believed in the past. It is a profound reconnection with yourself, which can spark the type of complete transformation you are here to create. Begin now.

Fertility Reset Prescription 6: The power of rebalancing your perspectives

Uncovering the benefits and drawbacks of having a baby is an essential step to ensure you are not romanticising something you want and don't yet have, and as a result causing yourself undue torment.

Dr John Demartini in his book *The Values Factor* presents a simple yet very effective exercise he uses to help people balance their perception.[11] I have adapted this exercise for my patients and now I share it with you. The wonderful thing about this exercise is that if you will do it – on paper (remember, cursive writing is the doing part of thinking and is vital for cognitive restructuring which of course is exactly what we are working towards here) – you will experience a kinesthetically based emotional transformation. In my opinion, this is one of the best exercises of its kind, if you choose to put in the minimal required effort. Merely thinking up some answers in your head just won't do in order to help you create the transformation you deserve. The good news is that if you will put the small effort to create these two lists, in a comparatively short amount of time you can transform your inner emotional world as it relates to every area of your life. Give your best to complete it, even if you do it in a few different sittings because it is the sheer mental 'weight lifting' of having to think up these many things that is capable of transforming your results.

Below or on a separate piece of paper you are to write down 200 drawbacks to having a baby and 200 benefits to not having one. And no, this is not a typo, the point of this exercise is to truly stretch your mind beyond what you think is possible and completely reshape your perspective. So, let's do this.

200 Drawbacks of Having a Baby	200 Benefits of NOT Having a Baby
1	1
2	2
3	3
4	4
5	5
6	6
7	7
8	8
9	9
10...	10...

If you have the willingness, courage and determination to truthfully answer my questions you will learn things about yourself and your situation you never knew or considered before. These two lists have the potential to completely transform your journey if you will allow it. As you did for Prescription 4, keep your lists handy so you can review them at least weekly for the first three months and then monthly until necessary.

You can also use this exercise in any other area of your life where a balanced perspective would be advantageous to you. For example: 200 benefits of having the worst boss in the world and 200 drawbacks to having the best boss in the world – the list of possibilities are truly endless. And you will be amazed at just how much better you will feel at having a fresh perspective of a previously 'horrible' situation once you actually discover all of the ways it serves you. You can still want to change it and improve it. In fact, it will become easier for you to do so because you will be less likely to come from a place of entitlement but rather a place of positive action towards the outcomes you want to create, and your entire life will benefit as a result.

Resources

There is a bonus transformational activity awaiting you in the book portal. Over the years of implementing it, I have seen people's world view change, but also a level of empowerment regarding their fertility journey that wasn't there before. I do know, however, that everyone who takes the time to go through these exercises I share eventually returns the favour and shares with me a story of metamorphosis that never fails to leave me with a tear of gratitude for the ability to introduce it to them.

Until now, I've only made these exercises available to patients in my clinic but I feel compelled to share it with you as well. So, go ahead and access the handout under Fertility Reset Prescription 6 in the interactive book portal now: http://thefertile.me/BreakthroughBook.

References

1   Schacter, D.L., et al., Memory distortion: an adaptive perspective. *Trends in Cognitive Sciences*, 2011. 15(10).

2   Sheldon, S., et al., A neurocognitive perspective on the forms and functions of autobiographical memory retrieval. *Frontiers in Systems Neuroscience*, 2019. 13.

3   Jonas, E., et al., Confirmation bias in sequential information search after preliminary decisions: An expansion of dissonance theoretical research on selective exposure to information. *Journal of Personality and Social Psychology*, 2001. 80(4).

4   Oprah Winfrey. *What I Know For Sure*. 2014, London, UK: Pan Macmillan.

5   Seligman, M., *Learned Optimism: How to Change Your Mind and Your Life*. 2006: Vintage.

6   Hasanpoor-Azghdy, S.B., et al., The emotional-psychological consequences of infertility among infertile women seeking treatment: Results of a qualitative study. *Iranian Journal of Reproductive Medicine*, 2014. 12(2).

7   Namdar, A., et al., Quality of life and general health of infertile women. *Health and Quality of Life Outcomes*, 2017. 15(1).

8   Patel, A., et al., Illness cognitions, anxiety, and depression in men and women undergoing fertility treatments: A dyadic approach. *Journal of Human Reproductive Sciences*, 2018. 11(2).

9   Seligman, M.E.P., et al., Positive psychotherapy. *The American Psychologist*, 2006. 61(8).

10   Seligman, M., *Helplessness: On Development, Depression, and Death*. 1975, New York: W.H. Freeman.

11   Dr J Demartini. *The Values Factor: The Secret to Creating an Inspired and Fulfilling Life*. 2013, US: Penguin Putnam.

CHAPTER 14

Prescription 7: Your Fertility X Factor Explained

'If you don't like something, change it; if you can't change it, change the way you think about it.'

Mary Engelbreit

O ur bodies didn't evolve to make reproduction their priority – survival has always been and continues to be paramount. When we're out of balance and in survival mode, even things that are ordinarily positive, such as receiving a promotion, more responsibility and a raise at work, can send the body's biochemistry into survival mode.

Balance is measured in degrees away from homeostasis. Any time you're doing too much or too little when it comes to sleep and exercise, your body's biochemistry swings from side to side, disrupting your homeostatic balance. This leads your body to behave very much like it did 10,000 years ago (when the main aim was to run away from the sabre-toothed tiger) when dealing with basic, day-to-day stress.

In survival mode, the body focuses all its energy and nutrient allocation towards the most important organs and systems that will help ward off immediate danger, and shuts down those that aren't essential to the task. The body has an internal conversation and decides that immune function isn't all that important during a fight-or-flight situation because the little bug inside isn't as much of a threat as the big, salivating monster outside. Digestion can also be shut down because, after all, if you're not running away, you'll soon become food – so never mind digesting any right now. And finally, the body asserts that the last priority is reproduction: shut that system down – permanently if necessary (is essentially what the body is thinking). The priority is survival, anything else is a mere inconvenience at this point.

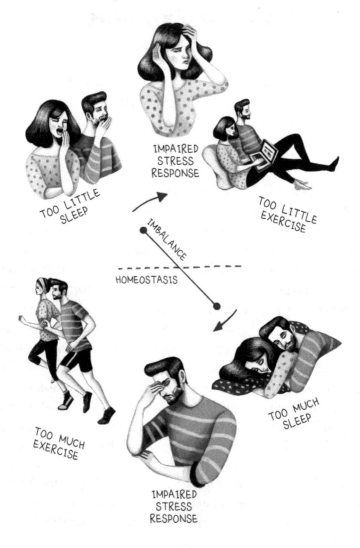

The body's aim is to focus on the shut-down systems once and if an opportunity arises. But due to the increasing demands placed on the body by our environments, poor food choices, stress and lack of sleep and movement, to name but a few of the obstacles, it hardly ever gets the chance to restore these systems to 100% capacity. Then add all that stressing about stress, and the fact that pregnancy is still nowhere to be seen, and you may continue to feed the imbalance. When we live in a continuous state of high alert, inadequately nourishing and nurturing ourselves, our reproductive organs don't receive the energy and nutrients they need to function optimally, particularly as we mature.

When a body (male or female) is out of balance, stress directly impacts its hormones and reproductive organs. It increases the production of cortisol, adrenaline and noradrenaline – also known as stress hormones.[1,2,3] The problem with this increase in stress hormone production is that reproductive hormones are made from the same precursor: pregnenolone.[4,5] So, it's easy to imagine what happens to reproductive function when too much of this hormone building block, pregnenolone, is being used to sustain the stress response instead of being channelled into effective reproductive function. High levels of stress hormones are associated with weight gain,[6,7,8] infertility[9,10,11] and miscarriage.[12,13,14,15]

In addition, male stress is shown to cause oxidative stress to sperm, which can lead to low sperm count, weakened sperm motility, fragmented DNA within the sperm cells and abnormally shaped sperm.[16,17,18,19,20] Stress is also associated with sexual dysfunction (eg impotence and ejaculation issues), which negatively impacts a couple's chances of conception and taking home a healthy baby.[21,22]

Excessive female stress can result in a cessation of both ovulation and menstruation.[11,23] It can negatively impact the biochemical and physical processes of egg maturation and release.[24,25] And stress can cause chemical changes and spasms in the fallopian tubes and uterus to prevent a fertilised egg from implanting.[26,27] It can also cause miscarriage after successful implantation.[28,29]

Unfortunately, couples faced with fertility issues often find themselves in a perpetually escalating stress-on-top-of-stress cycle. Stress increases the imbalance that continues to bring disappointment, month after month, and as a result the stress piles on further, continuing to hinder fertility. So, how do you break this exasperating cycle?

The simple answer is: don't isolate reproductive function as if it weren't part of a whole, integrated system, or treat it as if it's some kind of 'numbers game' or Russian roulette.

Holistically treating the body and mind is critical to increasing your chances of conception. In my clinic, we place as much focus on the mindset required to take charge of one's fertility as we do on the physical components of treating reproductive function because, as a part of a full and remarkable solution, it truly is the best way I have seen results for my patients, even after everything else had failed.

After all, it's your mindset that has the power to lift you to your highest potential or keep you going around in circles in despair. A finely tuned mindset is responsible for most of the commitment and motivation necessary to create lasting change. Change which is the core of helping couples overcome infertility and miscarriage.

MIRACLE MOMENTS

• THE CLOCK IS TICKING •
JIM AND JENNY

I gave birth to our first daughter three months before my thirty-fifth birthday. It had taken over two years to conceive, and three rounds of IVF. All that time I was worrying about the possibility of an early menopause because my mother went through menopause in her late thirties. We really wanted a larger family, and I felt there just wasn't time to waste and to wait for nature to take its course. When our daughter was six months old, we went back to IVF.

We tried everything we could think of and were advised to do – implemented advice from multiple IVF clinics, took herbs and supplements prescribed by a local naturopath, read every article on the internet, got treatment from an acupuncturist, underwent rounds of tests, including PGS testing, ate a completely vegan diet for one year, and went through another twenty, yes twenty (fully stimulated) rounds of IVF – yet I still didn't get pregnant.

We sought opinions from four different senior people in the IVF industry and they all told us that the only option was a few invasive procedures which might increase my ability to conceive by 1% or donor egg. In short, they told us there was nothing further they could do. The odds were too slim.

Fortunately, we came across Gabriela and our lives changed. Gabriela and her team did extensive consultations and tests and helped support us emotionally. We really needed someone on our side. Given the ticking menopause clock and the fact that we'd undertaken so many IVF procedures already, we were under incredible stress.

Gabriela's team suggested major lifestyle changes to reduce the stress, including a healthy eating regime. We implemented as many of the recommended changes in our day-to-day life as we could (giving up bread and pasta is hard for a half-Italian!), making our home chemical free, changing our cookware, exercising, etc – in addition to going through the most thorough testing protocol I'd ever experienced, despite over twenty failed IVF attempts! It was certainly not for the faint-hearted, but we felt that we were able to 'do' something to change our outcome.

The tests showed that I was suffering from adrenal insufficiency, likely as a result of the many challenges we had faced in the four preceding years, including infertility, serious financial difficulties, commencing a new business (the operation of two law firms), anxiety and looking after our daughter. I was exhausted, and my body was too.

We also discovered that my uterus receptivity was two days out from my actual cycle days.

Gabriela helped us change our mindset, and by removing some of the stressful situations, reorganising our business commitments and giving my body the chance to recover from the years of IVF treatments and stress, we started to feel relaxed and calm again.

Between Christmas and New Year, we finally took a well-deserved break and enjoyed a few stress-free date nights. On day thirty-five of my January cycle, I was speaking to my program practitioner and she urged me to take a pregnancy test. I never considered I could be pregnant, and I was shocked by the result. After four years of trying to conceive, twenty-four rounds of IVF in total, being told by several doctors there was nothing further they could do, and enormous sacrifice and determination, we got pregnant naturally. I was thirty-nine years old.

After our beautiful baby was born, there was a third addition to our family – I got pregnant again in my forties. A true testament to the effectiveness of our efforts and the work of Gabriela and her team.

To make strides in the right direction, we need to focus, as always, on the least possible effort for maximum results. In this case, we must minimise the swinging of your Homeostatic Fertility Pendulum™

by consistently applying everything we've looked at so far. And we must add to your efforts the two solid pillars of sleep and exercise from the 11 Pillars of Fertility Foundations™.

Refreshing and rejuvenating sleep

The benefits of sleep are far reaching. A good night's sleep will have you ready to conquer the world. A bad one will have you crawling on your knees, begging for the end of the week, or worse, searching for stimulants to keep you on your feet. Quality sleep improves brain function, memory recall and mood.[30] Consistently getting enough sleep will also boost immunity, help you live a longer, happier life,[31,32,33,34,35,36] and help to improve egg[37,38,39] and sperm quality.[40,41,42] In addition, sleep will improve hormonal balance, which in turn helps optimise reproductive and sexual function.[43,44,45,46] Better sleep will even make you a better lover.[47,48,49,50] And who knows, despite the trials of trying to get pregnant, you may even start to enjoy sex again. If only every other health intervention had this kind of side effect.

• WHY IS SLEEP SO IMPORTANT FOR REPRODUCTION? •

Sleep is one of the body's few (and crucial) opportunities to enhance hormonal and brain neurotransmitter biochemical balance.[51,52] This self-regulation is essential to overcoming fertility challenges.

Sleep is indispensable in helping to balance melatonin and all the other important brain chemicals, which help the body achieve homeostatic balance.[53,54,55]

As far as fertility is concerned, melatonin is an especially important hormone that peaks in the early part of the evening. This melatonin peak, essential for optimum sleep, health and fertility happens most effectively when you're already in a restful state and not while staring at backlit screens.[56,57]

Balanced melatonin levels, along with giving you a peaceful and restful sleep, have a direct positive impact on improving egg[58,59,60] and sperm quality.[61,62,63] So, it's safe to say your fertility depends on it. And although melatonin supplementation is available, naturally balancing this important hormone and all other neurotransmitters through getting enough sleep is the most ideal way to optimise your fertility (because of all the other benefits sleep brings).

When it comes to sleep, both quantity and quality count. Here are my top three tips for improving your sleep quality right away.

Top tip #1: Go to bed at the same time every day (yes, every day)

This helps to reset your body clock and enhance hormonal balance. This will work especially well when you're in bed by 9pm or 10pm – you give your body full opportunity to take advantage of the melatonin's peaking time.

If you aren't sleepy then, here's how you change this: get up at 5am every day (including weekends). You'll have no problems getting to bed 'on time'. This is one of the most crucial and highly effective steps in sleep hygiene. Consistency is key for optimum results.[64,65,66]

Top tip #2: Create your own oasis

Transform your bedroom into your special haven. First, do a massive decluttering exercise – get rid of anything you no longer need or shouldn't be there, and make sure that everything has a place and everything is put in its place. Second, unplug any electronic devices from power points. Electromagnetic paraphernalia in the bedroom, including TVs, computers, phones, waterbeds, electric blankets and even alarm clocks can disrupt the pineal gland and the production of melatonin, serotonin and other important hormones and neurotransmitters essential for optimum sleep quality, moods and fertility.[67,68] Radiation exposure can also have a direct negative impact on cellular health and damage the egg and sperm.[69,70,71,72,73] The key is to live an unplugged life during your sleep, at the very least.

Top tip #3: Don't engage in stimulating activities just before bed

Enforce a work curfew and stop working by 7pm whenever possible. It's ideal to have a two- or three-hour break from any mentally engaging activities before bedtime. And for some people, this includes watching television or reading that's too stimulating. Even exercise close to bedtime can be too stimulating. Research suggests that to avoid negatively impacting your sleep, you should finish exercising at least six hours before bed.[74,75]

Now, the answer to the ultimate question – how much sleep should you be getting? Different people need different amounts of sleep to feel completely rested, but the consensus among research institutes around the world is that seven to nine hours is the ideal for optimum health and, of course, fertility.[76,77,78]

Moving with life

'Those who think they have no time for bodily exercise
will sooner or later have to find time for illness.'

Edward Stanley

Exercise is the secret weapon that can change so much on your fertility journey. Conclusive scientific research spouts its numerous benefits, from improved brain function and circulation to hormonal, blood sugar and mood regulation and much more. Various recent studies even show that a healthy preconception diet and exercise interventions normalise the sperm DNA of obese fathers and improve the health of the offspring.[79,80,81,82] Need I say more? The same benefits apply to prospective mothers, too.[83,84,85,86]

On the other hand, too much of a good thing is never ideal. Excessive exercise can contribute to reproductive abnormalities and infertility in men and women.[87,88,89] The key? Find the middle ground. If you're a couch potato, you need to change that. If you're an athlete, you may need to adjust or even severely reduce your training and increase your body fat percentage if you want to have a baby and are experiencing difficulties.

The current exercise recommendation for peak fertility (and health) is sixty minutes of moderate exercise five to seven days per week.[90,91] Moderate is essentially 65% to 85% intensity of exertion.[88,92] You don't want to kill yourself in the process, but you certainly want to feel you're alive while exercising.

For men, it's ideal to avoid cycling altogether for optimum fertility due to increased risk of nerve damage, excessive pressure to the testicles, and heat, all of which damage sperm and negatively impact fertility,[93,94,95,96] also increasing the risk of developing impotence.[97,98] Swimming in chlorinated pools[99,100] and exercising near or on main roads[101,102,103] also work against optimum fertility for men and women.

Ensure you take exercise at your own pace. It's great to feel you're pushing yourself, but if you've just got off the couch, it's not a good idea to sign up for a marathon as your next 'getting active' step. (Not that I would recommend a marathon at any point during the preconception preparation period or conception-attempt stage, anyway.) Pace yourself, build up your ability and fitness slowly, but work at it daily. Or, at the very minimum, three to five times per week – especially if you're currently not doing much more than 'fork lifting' (as my mum likes to call it) and/or 'couch surfing'.

Some people take classes, others go to the gym or for brisk walks around the park. Whatever you like, pick something and 'just do it'. Personally, unless I have a trainer cracking the whip or I'm training with a buddy, I find the gym quite boring – but comfortable and most importantly *doable*. I take my audiobooks and end up looking forward to working out because I can find out what happens next in my book. The important thing is that the strategy gets me there. Whatever works for you, implement it – that's the key.

Above all, remember why you're doing this. Ultimately, you're doing it for yourself and for a better quality of life – now and in the future.

So, get out there and do your part to balance your Homeostatic Fertility Pendulum™ by getting enough sleep and enough exercise. Address the stress component as well, where necessary.

MIRACLE MOMENTS

• TAKING ON THE BEST OF BOTH WORLDS FOR A SUCCESSFUL OUTCOME •

MEGAN AND WAYNE

We'd been trying to conceive for around twelve months when we decided to get some tests done with our GP. We were happy when no clear issues were identified, but it also felt daunting – what next? I really didn't want to go down the IVF route and was sure that there was a more natural approach.

This was when I first came across Gabriela and the Natural Fertility Breakthrough Program™. I was excited that it appeared there was something else out there – and the results seemed to speak for themselves – but I had a hard time convincing my husband that another approach was a possibility. So, I agreed to follow our doctor's suggestion, starting with a highly regarded IVF specialist.

After some testing, it was concluded that my husband's sperm were perfect but that I had PCOS – a diagnosis that wouldn't exactly prevent us from conceiving but we were told would make it more difficult. I was keen to investigate the effects of diet, supplements, etc to improve the situation but was constantly told that these things would make no difference.

We agreed to start with six rounds of assisted IUI, but it was a long, drawn-out process of getting the dosage of meds right. After twelve months, we had completed only five IUI cycles and we were still not pregnant, but I had had enough at this stage, and we moved on to IVF.

We were shocked to discover that during the first round of IVF, we had a 0% fertilisation rate. We were advised to try again with ICSI to assist with getting the eggs fertilised, and this time we ended up with three day-three embryos. The first fresh transfer resulted in failed implantation. We then underwent a frozen embryo transfer (FET), and two weeks later, we returned a positive result. We were over the moon.

However, seven and a half weeks in, and less than twenty-four hours before our first scan, I miscarried. We were utterly devastated and felt so alone and helpless. We found comfort in knowing that we had another embryo in the freezer. We transferred the last of our embryos in another FET. Two weeks later, we returned a negative result.

We then undertook our second ICSI cycle, and this time our specialist wanted to take all fertilised embryos through to blastocyst stage (day five). The cycle started promising, with eight eggs being fertilised. By day three, we had five of the embryos still looking strong. But by day four, they were all starting to lag noticeably, and by day five, there were none left. All had regressed and we were left with a devastating 0% success rate. Our specialist explained that it was most likely an egg-quality issue and we should start looking for a donor egg. At this stage we parted ways and I decided that we needed to try something different.

I decided to revisit the idea of Gabriela's program and announced to my husband that I was completing the application to be a part of their next intake and that we'd take it from there. I'd been following Gabriela's work for years on Facebook and felt as though it aligned with the holistic lifestyle changes I'd been making over the last few years. To my surprise, he had no objections, and suddenly I felt that we were taking charge of our situation, and I felt empowered.

We attended an information session with Gabriela's team, where we were asked some pretty challenging questions. When we were accepted into the program, while I couldn't see the whole road ahead, just the first step we needed to take, I was ready to trust the process.

There were many changes in lifestyle and habits that neither of us saw coming, and although the learning curve felt overwhelming at the start, we held each other up when either of us slipped. Irrespective of the challenges we faced, we were going to give it 100% each because we knew that a baby is equal parts mother and father.

Approximately twelve months into program, we were feeling healthier than ever and started natural conception attempts. But my cycle was still having trouble regulating, even with mild drug therapy, and given our previously zero IVF fertilisation rate, we were aware that we might have to return to ICSI. So, along with the guidance of our program practitioner, we decided to find a new IVF specialist to work with. We all decided that it was worth trying to perform PGS on any blastocysts (assuming that we would even make it that far).

We kicked off our first ICSI cycle under the new specialist (our first since starting the Natural Fertility Breakthrough Program™) and low and behold, we were able to freeze one day-five embryo and one day-six embryo. Both embryos were grade two, which meant their cells were beautifully divided and they were robust. Tears of joy streamed down our face as we hung up the phone from the lab. We knew the results were due to what we'd been putting into practice with Gabriela's team.

We decided to embryo bank and in subsequent cycles, we had roughly the same number of eggs collected, and similar fertilisation rates as the first cycle. And after the third round, we'd made it to six embryos and were now able to have them biopsied for PGS testing. After a nervous seven-day wait, the lab confirmed that of the five that were tested, three were chromosomally normal, one was abnormal and had been discarded and one was technically a 'no result'.

In only two and a half years, we had gone from failing to get embryo development past day three to having three beautiful PGS-tested embryos ready to go.

It was evident to us that correcting the minor factors that were affecting egg, sperm and our overall health had been the difference. The Natural Fertility Breakthrough Program™ had been the difference.

Soon it became time to perform the first FET. After a nerve-wracking two-week wait, it finally came time to do the beta-hCG blood test. We were sitting at a local café when my mobile rang. It was the nursing staff from the clinic, and I instantly felt nauseous with anticipation. Surrounded by strangers at a wobbly café table, holding each other's hands tight, we heard, 'Congratulations, you're pregnant.'

Both my husband and I believe that without having taken the huge leap of faith and starting on the Natural Fertility Breakthrough Program™ with Gabriela and her team, we would be in a very different place today. We quite possibly might have given up on our dream of having children of our own. Now, after numerous failed IUI and IVF/ICSI cycles and attempts, our beautiful baby girl has finally graced our lives and, upon Gabriela's request, also the very cover of this book.

Breaking the vicious cycle of stress

The best way to begin making improvements in any area is to first get clear on what you want to achieve. In the case of stress management, this is followed by clearly identifying the sources creating undue pressure. Write them down. Make a list if you must. Once you know the sources, you'll have a better idea of how to approach them. Remember, you can apply the tools and exercises I've shared with you in Prescriptions 4 and 6 to every single area of your life. Here are some additional ways to put a spring in your step:

- Schedule your daily activities in a way that leaves you time to unwind at some point.

- While cleaning the house or cooking or just doing nothing, put on some music that heightens your mood or relaxes or soothes you (and your partner) and enjoy it.

- You don't have to be a professional masseuse – just the touch of hands is soothing, reassuring and a sensuous prelude to love (not baby) making, which can be a wonderful way to connect with your partner and decompress. A professional deep-tissue massage is also well worth it from time to time.

- Yoga is very effective for relieving stress. If you don't belong to a club or studio, download an app and enjoy a great class in the comfort of your own home.

- Carve out a quiet space in your day to silence mind chatter and do some deep breathing and meditating.

- Talk it out with a friend, and if you don't have a trusted friend on board to whom you can vent, it may be worth it to see a counsellor. Doing so may give you a fresh perspective.

- Eliminate caffeine. It can negatively impact both male[104,105] and female fertility[106,107,108,109,110] and is also often too stimulating for the adrenals, which are already working overtime during periods of stress.[111,112,113] Treat yourself to a relaxing herbal tea such as chamomile, lemongrass or passion flower.

- Think positive thoughts. If you keep telling yourself 'I'll never get pregnant', you'll buy into fear and become depressed. And then you'll be more likely to engage in behaviour that is less than optimal for your overall health and fertility. Replace that negative voice in your head with positive imagery.[114,115] Visualisation has been shown to have deeply effective physical benefits for fertility.[116,117,118] Be sure to focus your visualisation activities firmly on your *areas of influence* (ie behaviours within your control rather than getting pregnant or having a baby – focus instead on what you can do that will get closer to your desired outcome) for best results.

- A romantic getaway with your partner can rejuvenate your relationship. It doesn't have to cost a lot – it can even be in your own city. Simply enjoy each other.

- Laugh. The power of laughter is well documented. 'Medical clowning' even improves pregnancy rates in women undergoing IVF.[119] But really, why stop there? The beneficial effects of humour in terms of a great quality of life are well established. Be sure to purposefully seek out and create opportunities to have fun. Whatever you enjoy will be a great start, but I'll also take the liberty of suggesting game nights with friends – not only to create bonds and connections with others but also to have hard belly laughs. Just. Have. Fun.

Fertility Reset Prescription 7: Balancing out your Homeostatic Fertility Pendulum™

Get creative with this task. Take a picture of the number one thing you need to implement to edge you towards balance: the thing that will make everything else easier or unnecessary in terms of getting your sleep, exercise and stress into balance. You may even want to create an artistic representation of this. It could be a drawing, a painting, a collage – whatever you like. Just make it a powerful visual reminder to keep you on track and in touch with your why and what you want to create in your life.

Once you've finished your masterpiece, put it somewhere you'll see it every day – on your fridge or in your planner, or make it your screensaver or your phone's wallpaper – post a photo of it on Instagram, and tag me in it (@fertilitybreakthrough or @gabrielarosafertility). I'd love to see what you're up to.

Resources

As a bonus gift, you'll find my full *Better Sleep for Optimum Fertility Pocket Guide* in the book portal. Visit http://thefertile.me/BreakthroughBook for everything you need to implement to get an even better sleep tonight.

References

1   Akhter, S., et al., The impact of periconceptional maternal stress on fecundability. *Annals of Epidemiology*, 2016. 26(10).

2   Goldstein, D.S., Adrenal responses to stress. *Cellular and Molecular Neurobiology*, 2010. 30(8).

3   Nargund, V.H., Effects of psychological stress on male fertility. *Nature Reviews. Urology*, 2015. 12(7).

4   Locci, A., et al., Neurosteroid biosynthesis down-regulation and changes in GABAA receptor subunit composition: A biomarker axis in stress-induced cognitive and emotional impairment. *British Journal of Pharmacology*, 2017. 174(19).

5   Whirledge, S., et al., Glucocorticoids, stress, and fertility. *Minerva Endocrinologica*, 2010. 35(2).

6   Block, J.P., et al., Psychosocial stress and change in weight among US adults. *American Journal of Epidemiology*, 2009. 170(2).

7   Chao, A.M., et al., Stress, cortisol, and other appetite-related hormones: Prospective prediction of 6-month changes in food cravings and weight. *Obesity* (Silver Spring, Md.), 2017. 25(4).

8   van der Valk, E.S., et al., Stress and obesity: Are there more susceptible individuals? *Current Obesity Reports*, 2018. 7(2).

9   An, Y., et al., Relationship between psychological stress and reproductive outcome in women undergoing in vitro fertilization treatment: Psychological and neurohormonal assessment. *Journal of Assisted Reproduction and Genetics*, 2013. 30(1).

10 Balk, J., et al., The relationship between perceived stress, acupuncture, and pregnancy rates among IVF patients: A pilot study. *Complementary Therapies in Clinical Practice*, 2010. 16(3).

11 Schliep, K.C., et al., Perceived stress, reproductive hormones, and ovulatory function: A prospective cohort study. *Epidemiology* (Cambridge, Mass.), 2015. 26(2).

12 Bashour, H., et al., Psychological stress and spontaneous abortion. *International Journal of Gynaecology and Obstetrics: The Official Organ of the International Federation of Gynaecology and Obstetrics*, 2001. 73(2).

13 Fenster, L., et al., Psychologic stress in the workplace and spontaneous abortion. *American Journal of Epidemiology*, 1995. 142(11).

14 Parker, V.J., et al., Stress in early pregnancy: Maternal neuro-endocrine-immune responses and effects. *Journal of Reproductive Immunology*, 2010. 85(1).

15 Qu, F., et al., The association between psychological stress and miscarriage: A systematic review and meta-analysis. *Scientific Reports*, 2017. 7.

16   Ilacqua, A., et al., Lifestyle and fertility: The influence of stress and quality of life on male fertility. *Reproductive Biology and Endocrinology: RB&E*, 2018. 16(1).

17   Janevic, T., et al., Effects of work and life stress on semen quality. *Fertility and Sterility*, 2014. 102(2).

18   Jurewicz, J., et al., The effect of stress on the semen quality. *Medycyna Pracy*, 2010. 61(6).

19   Radwan, M., et al., Sperm DNA damage – the effect of stress and everyday life factors. *International Journal of Impotence Research*, 2016. 28(4).

20   Zorn, B., et al., Psychological factors in male partners of infertile couples: Relationship with semen quality and early miscarriage. *International Journal of Andrology*, 2008. 31(6).

21   Barata, B.C., Affective disorders and sexual function: From neuroscience to clinic. *Current Opinion in Psychiatry*, 2017. 30(6).

22   Kalaitzidou, I., et al., Stress management and erectile dysfunction: A pilot comparative study. *Andrologia*, 2014. 46(6).

23   Michopoulos, V., et al., Neuroendocrine recovery initiated by cognitive behavioral therapy in women with functional hypothalamic amenorrhea: A randomized controlled trial. *Fertility and Sterility*, 2013. 99(7).

24   Tiwari, M., et al., Involvement of reactive oxygen species in meiotic cell cycle regulation and apoptosis in mammalian oocytes. *Reactive Oxygen Species*, 2016. 1(2).

25   Prasad, S., et al., Impact of stress on oocyte quality and reproductive outcome. *Journal of Biomedical Science*, 2016. 23.

26   Nepomnaschy, P.A., et al., Stress and female reproductive function: A study of daily variations in cortisol, gonadotrophins, and gonadal steroids in a rural Mayan population. *American Journal of Human Biology: The Official Journal of the Human Biology Council*, 2004. 16(5).

27   Nepomnaschy, P.A., et al., Cortisol levels and very early pregnancy loss in humans. *Proceedings of the National Academy of Sciences of the United States of America*, 2006. 103(10).

28   Field, T., et al., Cortisol: The culprit prenatal stress variable. *The International Journal of Neuroscience*, 2008. 118(8).

29   González-Ochoa, R., et al., Evaluating stress during pregnancy: Do we have the right conceptions and the correct tools to assess it? *Journal of Pregnancy*, 2018.

30   Goldstein, A.N., et al., The role of sleep in emotional brain function. *Annual Review of Clinical Psychology*, 2014. 10.

31   Domínguez, F., et al., Association of sleep duration and quality with subclinical atherosclerosis. *Journal of the American College of Cardiology*, 2019. 73(2).

32 Lovato, N., et al., Insomnia and mortality: A meta-analysis. *Sleep Medicine Reviews*, 2019. 43.

33 Mazzotti, D.R., et al., Human longevity is associated with regular sleep patterns, maintenance of slow wave sleep, and favorable lipid profile. *Frontiers in Aging Neuroscience*, 2014. 6.

34 Musiek, E.S., et al., Mechanisms linking circadian clocks, sleep, and neurodegeneration. *Science* (New York, N.Y.), 2016. 354(6315).

35 Shin, J.-e., et al., How a good sleep predicts life satisfaction: The role of zero-sum beliefs about happiness. *Frontiers in Psychology*, 2018. 9.

36 Steptoe, A., et al., Positive affect, psychological well-being, and good sleep. *Journal of Psychosomatic Research*, 2008. 64(4).

37 Goldstein, C.A., et al., Sleep in women undergoing in vitro fertilization: A pilot study. *Sleep Medicine*, 2017. 32.

38 Lin, Y.-H., et al., Somatic symptoms, sleep disturbance and psychological distress among women undergoing oocyte pick-up and in vitro fertilisation-embryo transfer. *Journal of Clinical Nursing*, 2016. 25(11-12).

39 Voiculescu, S.E., et al., Role of melatonin in embryo fetal development. *Journal of Medicine and Life*, 2014. 7(4).

40 Liu, M.-M., et al., Sleep deprivation and late bedtime impair sperm health through increasing antisperm antibody production: A prospective study of 981 healthy men. *Medical Science Monitor: International Medical Journal of Experimental and Clinical Research*, 2017. 23.

41 Palnitkar, G., et al., Linking sleep disturbance to idiopathic male infertility. *Sleep Medicine Reviews*, 2018. 42.

42 Viganò, P., et al., Sleep disturbances and semen quality in an Italian cross sectional study. *Basic and Clinical Andrology*, 2017. 27.

43 Andersen, M.L., et al., The association of testosterone, sleep, and sexual function in men and women. *Brain Research*, 2011. 1416.

44 Cho, J.W., et al., Sleep, sleep disorders, and sexual dysfunction. *The World Journal of Men's Health*, 2018.

45 Goldstein, C.A., et al., Sleep, circadian rhythms, and fertility. *Current Sleep Medicine Reports*, 2016. 2(4).

46 White, N.D., Influence of sleep on fertility in women. *American Journal of Lifestyle Medicine*, 2016. 10(4).

47 Kalmbach, D.A., et al., The impact of sleep on female sexual response and behavior: A pilot study. *The Journal of Sexual Medicine*, 2015. 12(5).

48 Kellesarian, S.V., et al., Association between obstructive sleep apnea and erectile dysfunction: A systematic review and meta-analysis. *International Journal of Impotence Research*, 2018. 30(3).

49   Maranges, H.M., et al., The rested relationship: Sleep benefits marital evaluations. *Journal of Family Psychology: JFP: Journal of the Division of Family Psychology of the American Psychological Association* (Division 43), 2017. 31(1).

50   Richter, K., et al., Two in a bed: The influence of couple sleeping and chronotypes on relationship and sleep. An overview. *Chronobiology International*, 2016. 33(10).

51   Clinton, J.M., et al., Biochemical regulation of sleep and sleep biomarkers. *Journal of Clinical Sleep Medicine: JCSM: Official Publication of the American Academy of Sleep Medicine*, 2011. 7(Suppl 5).

52   Kim, T.W., et al., The impact of sleep and circadian disturbance on hormones and metabolism. *International Journal of Endocrinology*, 2015. 2015.

53   Holst, S.C., et al., Sleep homeostasis, metabolism, and adenosine. *Current Sleep Medicine Reports*, 2015. 1(1).

54   Longordo, F., et al., Consequences of sleep deprivation on neurotransmitter receptor expression and function. *The European Journal of Neuroscience*, 2009. 29(9).

55   Oh, J., et al., The role of co-neurotransmitters in sleep and wake regulation. *Molecular Psychiatry*, 2018.

56   Nagendra, R.P., et al., Meditation and its regulatory role on sleep. *Frontiers in Neurology*, 2012. 3.

57   Pandi-Perumal, S.R., et al., Melatonin: Nature's most versatile biological signal? *The FEBS Journal*, 2006. 273(13).

58   Jahromi, B.N., et al., Effect of melatonin on the outcome of assisted reproductive technique cycles in women with diminished ovarian reserve: A double-blinded randomized clinical trial. *Iranian Journal of Medical Sciences*, 2017. 42(1).

59   Kim, M.K., et al., Does supplementation of in-vitro culture medium with melatonin improve IVF outcome in PCOS? *Reproductive Biomedicine Online*, 2013. 26(1).

60   Tamura, H., et al., Melatonin and the ovary: Physiological and pathophysiological implications. *Fertility and Sterility*, 2009. 92(1).

61   Bejarano, I., et al., Exogenous melatonin supplementation prevents oxidative stress-evoked DNA damage in human spermatozoa. *Journal of Pineal Research*, 2014. 57(3).

62   Li, C., et al., Melatonin and male reproduction. *Clinica Chimica Acta; International Journal of Clinical Chemistry*, 2015. 446.

63   Najafi, A., et al., Melatonin affects membrane integrity, intracellular reactive oxygen species, caspase3 activity and AKT phosphorylation in frozen thawed human sperm. *Cell and Tissue Research*, 2018. 372(1).

64   Burgess, H.J., et al., A late wake time phase delays the human dim light melatonin rhythm. *Neuroscience Letters*, 2006. 395(3).

65   Goel, N., et al., Circadian rhythms, sleep deprivation, and human performance. *Progress in Molecular Biology and Translational Science*, 2013. 119.

66   Sharma, M.P., et al., Behavioral interventions for insomnia: Theory and practice. *Indian Journal of Psychiatry*, 2012. 54(4).

67   Gooley, J.J., et al., Exposure to room light before bedtime suppresses melatonin onset and shortens melatonin duration in humans. *The Journal of Clinical Endocrinology and Metabolism*, 2011. 96(3).

68   Shochat, T., Impact of lifestyle and technology developments on sleep. *Nature and Science of Sleep*, 2012. 4.

69   Adams, J.A., et al., Effect of mobile telephones on sperm quality: A systematic review and meta-analysis. *Environment International*, 2014. 70.

70   Kesari, K.K., et al., Radiations and male fertility. *Reproductive Biology and Endocrinology: RB&E*, 2018. 16.

71   Kıvrak, E.G., et al., Effects of electromagnetic fields exposure on the antioxidant defense system. *Journal of Microscopy and Ultrastructure*, 2017. 5(4).

72   Roozbeh, N., et al., Influence of radiofrequency electromagnetic fields on the fertility system: Protocol for a systematic review and meta-analysis. *JMIR Research Protocols*, 2018. 7(2).

73   Santini, S.J., et al., Role of mitochondria in the oxidative stress induced by electromagnetic fields: Focus on reproductive systems. *Oxidative Medicine and Cellular Longevity*, 2018. 2018.

74   Dolezal, B.A., et al., Interrelationship between sleep and exercise: A systematic review. *Advances in Preventive Medicine*, 2017. 2017.

75   Fairbrother, K., et al., Effects of exercise timing on sleep architecture and nocturnal blood pressure in prehypertensives. *Vascular Health and Risk Management*, 2014. 10.

76   Chen, Q., et al., Inverse U-shaped association between sleep duration and semen quality: Longitudinal observational study (MARHCS) in Chongqing, China. *Sleep*, 2016. 39(1).

77   Kloss, J.D., et al., Sleep, sleep disturbance and fertility in women. *Sleep Medicine Reviews*, 2015. 22.

78   Watson, N.F., et al., Joint consensus statement of the American academy of sleep medicine and sleep research society on the recommended amount of sleep for a healthy adult: Methodology and discussion. *Sleep*, 2015. 38(8).

79   Al Omrani, B., et al., Associations of sperm DNA fragmentation with lifestyle factors and semen parameters of Saudi men and its impact on ICSI outcome. *Reproductive Biology and Endocrinology: RB&E*, 2018. 16.

80   Houfflyn, S., et al., Male obesity: Epigenetic origin and effects in sperm and offspring. *Current Molecular Biology Reports*, 2017. 3(4).

81   Mir, J., et al., Impact of weight loss on sperm DNA integrity in obese men. *Andrologia*, 2018.

82   Oliveira, J.B.A., et al., Association between body mass index and sperm quality and sperm DNA integrity. A large population study. *Andrologia*, 2018. 50(3).

83   Best, D., et al., How effective are weight-loss interventions for improving fertility in women and men who are overweight or obese? A systematic review and meta-analysis of the evidence. *Human Reproduction Update*, 2017. 23(6).

84   Gaskins, A.J., et al., Prepregnancy nutrition and early pregnancy outcomes. *Current Nutrition Reports*, 2015. 4(3).

85   Panth, N., et al., The influence of diet on fertility and the implications for public health nutrition in the United States. *Frontiers in Public Health*, 2018. 6.

86   van Oers, A.M., et al., Effectiveness of lifestyle intervention in subgroups of obese infertile women: A subgroup analysis of a RCT. *Human Reproduction* (Oxford, England), 2016. 31(12).

87   Gordon, C.M., et al., Functional hypothalamic amenorrhea: An Endocrine Society clinical practice guideline. *The Journal of Clinical Endocrinology and Metabolism*, 2017. 102(5).

88   Hakimi, O., et al., Effect of exercise on ovulation: A systematic review. *Sports Medicine* (Auckland, N.Z.), 2017. 47(8).

89   Tartibian, B., et al., Correlation between seminal oxidative stress biomarkers and antioxidants with sperm DNA damage in elite athletes and recreationally active men. *Clinical Journal of Sport Medicine: Official Journal of the Canadian Academy of Sport Medicine*, 2012. 22(2).

90   WHO, Global recommendations on physical activity for health.

91   Russo, L.M., et al., A prospective study of physical activity and fecundability in women with a history of pregnancy loss. *Human Reproduction* (Oxford, England), 2018. 33(7).

92   Thomson, R.L., et al., The effect of a hypocaloric diet with and without exercise training on body composition, cardiometabolic risk profile,and reproductive function in overweight and obese women with polycystic ovary syndrome. *The Journal of Clinical Endocrinology & Metabolism*, 2008. 93(9).

93   Hajizadeh Maleki, B., et al., Long-term low-to-intensive cycling training: Impact on semen parameters and seminal cytokines. *Clinical Journal of Sport Medicine: Official Journal of the Canadian Academy of Sport Medicine*, 2015. 25(6).

94   Ibañez-Perez, J., et al., An update on the implication of physical activity on semen quality: A systematic review and meta-analysis. *Archives of Gynecology and Obstetrics*, 2019.

95   Panara, K., et al., Adverse effects of common sports and recreational activities on male reproduction. *European Urology Focus*, 2018.

96   Jozkow, P., et al., The impact of intense exercise on semen quality. *American Journal of Mens Health*, 2017. 11(3).

97   Papagiannopoulos, D., et al., Evaluation of young men with organic erectile dysfunction. *Asian Journal of Andrology*, 2015. 17(1).

98   Sommer, F., et al., Bicycle riding and erectile dysfunction: A review. *The Journal of Sexual Medicine*, 2010. 7(7).

99   Manasfi, T., et al., Occurrence, origin, and toxicity of disinfection byproducts in chlorinated swimming pools: An overview. *International Journal of Hygiene and Environmental Health*, 2017. 220(3).

100   Nickmilder, M., et al., Associations between testicular hormones at adolescence and attendance at chlorinated swimming pools during childhood. *International Journal of Andrology*, 2011. 34(5 Pt 2).

101   Carré, J., et al., Does air pollution play a role in infertility?: A systematic review. *Environmental Health: A Global Access Science Source*, 2017. 16(1).

102   Mahalingaiah, S., et al., Adult air pollution exposure and risk of infertility in the Nurses' Health Study II. *Human Reproduction* (Oxford, England), 2016. 31(3).

103   Qin, F., et al., Exercise and air pollutants exposure: A systematic review and meta-analysis. *Life Sciences*, 2019. 218.

104   Karmon, A.E., et al., Male caffeine and alcohol intake in relation to semen parameters and in vitro fertilization outcomes among fertility patients. *Andrology*, 2017. 5(2).

105   Ricci, E., et al., Coffee and caffeine intake and male infertility: A systematic review. *Nutrition Journal*, 2017. 16(1).

106   Lyngsø, J., et al., Association between coffee or caffeine consumption and fecundity and fertility: A systematic review and dose-response meta-analysis. *Clinical Epidemiology*, 2017. 9.

107   Oostingh, E.C., et al., The impact of maternal lifestyle factors on periconception outcomes: A systematic review of observational studies. *Reproductive Biomedicine Online*, 2019. 38(1).

108   Peacock, A., et al., Adherence to the caffeine intake guideline during pregnancy and birth outcomes: A prospective cohort study. *Nutrients*, 2018. 10(3).

109   Rosa, G., 'How caffeine impacts fertility when trying to conceive.' 2019. Retrieved from https://naturalfertilitybreakthrough.com/infographics.

110   Lane, J.D., et al., Caffeine affects cardiovascular and neuroendocrine activation at work and home. *Psychosomatic Medicine*, 2002. 64(4).

111   Lovallo, W.R., et al., Stress-like adrenocorticotropin responses to caffeine in young healthy men. *Pharmacology, Biochemistry, and Behavior*, 1996. 55(3).

112   Lovallo, W.R., et al., Cortisol responses to mental stress, exercise, and meals following caffeine intake in men and women. *Pharmacology, Biochemistry, and Behavior*, 2006. 83(3).

113   Lovallo, W.R., et al., Caffeine may potentiate adrenocortical stress responses in hypertension-prone men. *Hypertension* (Dallas, Tex.: 1979), 1989. 14(2).

114   Bleil, M.E., et al., Fertility treatment response: Is it better to be more optimistic or less pessimistic? *Psychosom Med*, 2012. 74(2).

115   Moeenizadeh, M., et al., The efficacy of well-being therapy for depression in infertile women. *International Journal of Fertility & Sterility*, 2017. 10(4).

116   Hosaka, T., et al., Effect of psychiatric group intervention on natural-killer cell activity and pregnancy rate. *General Hospital Psychiatry*, 2002. 24(5).

117   Jallo, N., et al., Guided imagery for stress and symptom management in pregnant African American women. *Evidence-based Complementary and Alternative Medicine: eCAM*, 2014. 2014.

118   Rooney, K.L., et al., The relationship between stress and infertility. *Dialogues in Clinical Neuroscience*, 2018. 20(1).

119   Friedler, S., et al., The effect of medical clowning on pregnancy rates after in vitro fertilization and embryo transfer. *Fertility and Sterility*, 2011. 95(6).

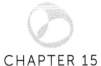

CHAPTER 15

Prescription 8: Understanding The Numbers Behind Your Test Results

'Optimism is the faith that leads to achievement.
Nothing can be done without hope and confidence.'

Helen Keller

I think it's easy for us to agree that a person is infinitely more than a collection of cells, or numbers on a piece of paper. But when it comes to fertility, two people are often reduced to these very things. I'm all for high tech, but not at the expense of patients being taught self-advocacy that's based on scientific evidence.

From a humane and public health standpoint, patients deserve better than the existing seventeen-year knowledge gap that arises from the time it takes scientific findings to filter into mainstream understanding.[1] This amount of time is already on the upper limit for most couples trying to conceive.

Those working to overcome infertility and miscarriage, especially people who have been trying to have a baby for over two years, deserve much more than they currently receive through standard fertility treatment. Patients experiencing extended time to baby deserve individualised, considered and personalised care, which only a change in the current medical practice paradigm can fulfil.

This is why I began working towards a master's in public health at Harvard University. I would like to continue contributing to the change I envision for patients we treat across the globe and millions more people like them.

There's still much work to be done, but this book and my work with patients over the last two decades are a couple of early seeds. Because frankly, 'your eggs are no good' and 'it's a numbers game' without any further assessment or interest in fine tuning and improving an individual's or a couple's situation to me, is simply unacceptable. Especially when this road is as long and hard as it is for so many. And when couples are thoroughly drained of their financial and emotional resources with nothing – not even improved health or emotional resilience – to show for their efforts. Science may hold the promise of endless possibility and captivating inquiry, but without empathy, love, compassion and real care for the person it's meant to serve, in my opinion, it fails its ultimate purpose: uplifting humanity.

Due to lack of support and appropriate guidance, many couples become desperate and give up sooner than they would have otherwise. On face value, this may not seem like a big problem in an already seemingly over-populated world, but such deep disappointments have in many instances the power to change life's trajectory. In time, some people may eventually turn these challenges into positives, although a vast portion of individuals who walk this path simply don't have the skills and necessary knowledge (or the opportunity for access to support) in order to make a positive meaning out of their personal tragedies. The resulting inability to effectively process these types of life circumstances can contribute to all sorts of mental health adversities, which can further lead people to engage in self-destructive behaviours.[2,3,4,5] Thus, the associated (physical, emotional and financial) costs of the lack of an integrative medical strategy ends up being much greater than individuals, families, and entire health care systems initially anticipate or account for.[6,7,8,9,10]

On these and many other points it is true that our patients differ greatly from the general population. So much so that I have now come to expect my patients to regularly defy the dire prognoses they'd previously been sentenced with through their similarly difficult journeys – sometimes against all odds. Maybe there is a lot to be said for a health bias, or maybe it's the confluence of their steadfastness of spirit, determination and effort in combination with guidance, accountability and emotional support that makes the ultimate difference. Regardless, my assessment of the net result based on the more than twenty years since I began this journey has long proven that 'immutable' numbers on a piece of paper or a computer screen are no match for what's possible when science, self-belief and the right strategy (and maybe even a little faith in brighter days) powerfully converge.

Unhelpful or insensitive remarks from a medical team can rob patients of the motivation required to do their best – for themselves. You may have personally experienced this type of situation. But make no mistake: hope and self-belief are crucial ingredients in helping you transform your results.[11,12]

Lest I be misunderstood, this isn't about false hope. In fact, if anything, I'm often accused by my patients of being a loving straight shooter who tells them what they need to hear rather than what they'd prefer to hear (always with the utmost love and respect for them and their situation). But if your belief is that nothing you do will be of use, you're sentencing yourself to a self-fulfilling prophecy. If you do nothing to change your circumstances, they will indeed remain exactly the same.

I'm all for deep-diving into high-tech diagnostics to aid in understanding the reasons a couple may be struggling to conceive. This approach can help guide better clinical decisions. But by no means are numbers on a piece of paper the only determinant of a couple's ability to overcome their challenge. Just because someone's assays may show a lower-than-ideal ovarian reserve, poor sperm parameters, or a need to improve egg quality, it doesn't mean they'll never have a baby. So in my clinic, we use the results of a constantly evolving, comprehensive fertility-testing protocol to learn where we stand and what we might be able to do about it, irrespective of a couple's prognosis elsewhere. We do this for two main reasons. Firstly, because their results help us understand what we need to *do* to optimise a couple's situation. Secondly, because we are impartial about what our patients may need to do to take home their healthy babies. We will make the most direct-line recommendation for a couple once we understand the obstacles in their way and have properly addressed said obstacles.

In every instance, we will make our recommendation and take our patients' cues as to when a change in strategy is necessary to get them to their outcome. Once there is true understanding and proper clarity, then and only then are we closer to a satisfactory outcome. This approach liberates people to make choices they would have never otherwise considered because they were stuck in erroneous thinking, going around in circles looking for answers.

To me and my team, a systematic and methodical process is everything. I want my patients to know we've left no stone unturned, so they can finally move forward and closer to their dream. I want my patients to exercise the power of choice regarding their fertility rather than fall victim to a circumstance. This is the path to real results.

It's all too easy to be fooled by looking at laboratory results. So, take it with a great big pinch of salt when anyone makes a pronouncement about your fertility (including likely chances of success or lack thereof based on them). The mere fact you're reading this book makes you different from the general population, from which many of the generally touted fertility statistics are extracted from.

Prevalence and incidence of infertility and miscarriage rates are extracted from general-population data. You just need to look around to see the declining state of health of the general population to uncover some alarming associations regarding reproductive choice, challenges and possible future outcomes around the globe. Given the status quo, it is also impossible to miss the fact that uncommon success typically follows uncommon behaviour. So, before you compare yourself on basic terms or allow the practitioner in charge of your case to make this mistake for you, be sure to dissect all the relevant facts. My patients are proof that just because two people are the same age or have a similar medical history or diagnosis, it doesn't necessarily follow that their outcomes will be the same after our intervention. This is especially true when a full understanding of a couple's obstacles remain improperly unexplored. Case in point: the 'unexplained infertility' diagnosis.

I've lost count of the number of times (in the thousands, for sure) I've sat with couples who have tried many different interventions without success but have had only the most basic of biochemical assessments (with the male typically having had many fewer or even none).

Optimum thyroid function

Here's a simple but pertinent example of this issue. It applies directly to the standard fertility workup most couples receive. Optimum thyroid function is of paramount importance when it comes to fertility. The big problem here is that for the most part, when a couple shows up for a discussion regarding difficulty getting pregnant, not much is asked about their general health. Often only the bare minimum is investigated, and then IVF/ICSI is proposed. At the next office, (sometimes) a few more basic examinations may be requested, and typically the discussion doesn't extend much further than determining when injections will begin and when to show up for monitoring throughout the cycle.

If the result of a single thyroid function parameter requested (take for example the thyroid stimulating hormone (TSH) parameter range 0.1 to 4 mU/L) returns as, say, 2.75 mU/L, it's simply pronounced 'within range' – even though many international fertility societies recommend that any result above 2.5 mU/L (in a woman trying to conceive) requires further assessment or at least monitoring but very likely treatment, particularly in cases of extended infertility and/or recurrent miscarriage.[13] Unfortunately, subclinical hypothyroidism often isn't even mentioned to the patient. The conversation about possible thyroid involvement is put to rest before it begins. Beyond, the commonly demonstrated suboptimal TSH result, which is often coupled with a history of miscarriage and even the possibility of thyroid-related implantation failure following IUI, IVF or ICSI, is also much more likely to occur if this issue is not addressed.[13,14,15,16]

This is why we look at our patients' cases from a holistic lens considering much more than just one single biochemical marker. I believe our patients deserve more from us than an incomplete assessment or an unexplained label.

MIRACLE MOMENTS

• AGAINST ALL ODDS •
HELENA AND TIM

After a year of trying to conceive naturally, we were told by a fertility specialist that my husband's sperm was not good and that there was absolutely nothing we could do other than try IVF. Thinking that at least we now knew why we were not getting pregnant, we jumped into our first IVF cycle with lots of hope.

I got twelve eggs at the retrieval, only four fertilised with ICSI. We decided to transfer one embryo and freeze the remaining three, but none of them made it to day five, so we had nothing to freeze. Two weeks later I got a BFN (Big Fat Negative). We were absolutely devastated.

Five months later, we decided to go for round two. Again twelve eggs were retrieved and four fertilised. I decided to transfer three embryos and leave one to freeze. Unfortunately, again, the remaining embryo didn't make it to day five, so we had nothing to freeze. Two weeks later I got BFN once more. We were really shocked that it didn't work. The doctor had no answers. I started to question everything. I was done with that clinic and decided to take a break and do some research.

This was around the time that I came across Gabriela, who was a speaker in a fertility summit. But I wasn't quite ready for Gabriela yet.

Two years after our second IVF attempt, we decided to find a new IVF clinic and try one more round. Our new doctor was interested in immunological testing. They retrieved eleven eggs, four fertilised with ICSI, and this time we also did PGS testing. Two out of the four embryos were normal. I couldn't do the fresh embryo transfer because my uterine lining was very thin, so I had to wait two more months. We transferred two embryos and again it resulted in a BFN.

The doctor told us that without donor eggs and probably a surrogate I would never get pregnant, that we should give up and adopt. I never saw him again.

I thought that egg donor was the only way for us to go, so I made an appointment at a third IVF clinic to discuss our options. At that point I came across Gabriela again and did one of her online programs. I was on board 100%, but the problem was my husband. He was sure that because IVF hadn't worked, doing things naturally wouldn't work. So, another year and a half went by but finally he agreed and about another year and a half later we officially started Gabriela's program.

After lots of comprehensive testing, we were prescribed supplements and herbal medicines based on our results, and we started to see improvements. My husband lost sixty pounds in five months, and I lost twenty-four pounds. He said he'd never felt better. And after we'd been on the program for five months, my husband's semen analysis results were completely normal. I had lots of problems – by this time, high FSH levels, low AMH levels, high oestrogen, thin uterine lining, adrenal fatigue, elevated natural killer cells and so on. But gradually my results started to improve as well, and we were soon ready to start trying naturally.

Amazingly, we were successful on our first attempt, but sadly, we lost the pregnancy at nine weeks because of chromosomal abnormalities. As much as it was heartbreaking for us, we now had hope again. We'd been told that we could never conceive without donor eggs and surrogacy, but we now knew that we could get pregnant naturally.

We took a break for a few months with the team's continued support, then on the second try we were pregnant again. This time, everything was perfect. Our baby boy, Tyler Jan, was born weighing ten pounds, two ounces. He's a very happy and healthy toddler. When he was four months old, we decided to join the program again and try for baby number two. I was already forty years old at that time, so we didn't want to wait too long. After being on the program for four months, we got pregnant again on a first attempt. Natalia Gabriela was born on Valentine's Day, weighing ten pounds, four ounces.

Now our family is complete, and we couldn't be happier. When I look at my babies, I have tears in my eyes because I never thought I would have even one baby, let alone two. I owe everything to Gabriela and her team.

What are the signs your thyroid could be malfunctioning? Both clinical and subclinical hyperthyroidism and/or hypothyroidism can negatively impact fertility and the ability to take a healthy pregnancy to term. Therefore, it's vital that this important yet often neglected fertility factor is assessed and monitored throughout your fertility journey (for both prospective parents because thyroid dysfunction also leads to sperm abnormalities as well).[17,18,19,20]

Thyroid Dysfunction

When investigating thyroid dysfunction, it's important to consider clinical symptomatology as well as laboratory findings. Here are some of my considerations when addressing both prospective parents.

HYPERTHYROIDISM

Table 6.1: Symptoms that characterise hyperthyroidism (overactive thyroid gland)

Common	Less common
• Heart palpitations, fast pulse and irregular heartbeat • Trembling and twitches • Heat intolerance • Hot flushes and increased sweating • Increased appetite (or loss of appetite) • Unintentional weight loss • Diarrhoea • Anxiety, nervousness and/or panic attacks • Restlessness • Irritability • Thin, moist skin • Soft, thinning hair • Shortness of breath • Muscle weakness • Insomnia	• Bowel disorders • Brittle nails • Chest pain • Cramps • Decreased libido • Easy bruising • Hair loss • Headaches and migraines • Sore throat • Swelling of legs • Other

[continued]

Common	Less Common
• Enlarged thyroid gland • Eye complaints (especially gritty or bulging eyes) • Fatigue, exhaustion and lack of energy • Menstrual-cycle disturbances (intermittent and light) • Infertility • Depression and mood swings	

HYPOTHYROIDISM

Hypothyroidism has been called the 'unsuspected illness', and it's frequently misdiagnosed.

Table 6.2: Symptoms that characterise hypothyroidism (underactive thyroid gland)

Common	Less common
• Weight gain • Chronic constipation • Feeling cold (especially hands and feet), even on warm days • Low BBT • Fatigue, exhaustion and low energy (even after twelve hours of sleep) • Slow reflexes • Slow, weak pulse • Slowness of thought processes (brain fog) • Indecisiveness • Poor memory and concentration • Sluggishness • Muscle weakness • Pain and stiffness in muscles or joints • Deepening, hoarse voice • Depression, mood swings and severe PMS	• Allergies • Back pain • Blood pressure problems • Breast tenderness • Irregular heartbeat • Chest pain • Digestive disturbances • Dizziness • Dry eyes and mouth • Headaches and migraines • Irritability • Pale skin • Heart palpitations • Reduced libido • Skin rashes • Sore throat

[continued]

Common	Less common
• Thick, dry, coarse skin • Creviced, cracking skin on heels, elbows and kneecaps • Enlarged thyroid gland • Lump in throat (hard to swallow) • High cholesterol • Menstrual-cycle irregularities (prolonged and heavy) • Infertility • Numbness and tingling (especially in hands and face) • Fluid retention (swelling of face and feet) • Brittle hair and nails • Hair loss • Shortness of breath on exertion	• Stiff neck and shoulders • Thinning eyebrows • Visual disturbances • Other

Not everyone has all these symptoms. You may relate to only a few, or you may relate to many. But if you're experiencing a combination of the above symptoms or suspect a thyroid problem, further testing is required.

A person suffering from either an overactive or underactive thyroid gland may find it difficult to cope with the symptoms from day to day. The pressure on bodily functions will continue to mount unless appropriate treatment is given.

MIRACLE MOMENTS

• IT'S A LONG TIME
TO KEEP HOPE ALIVE •
THE STORY OF GRETA AND MATTHEW

I had been diagnosed with polycystic ovarian syndrome and was suffering from irregular and sometimes missing menstrual periods and finding it difficult to lose weight and get pregnant. After visiting naturopaths and trying lots of natural and conventional therapies to get pregnant, without success, I was despondent. All the medical professionals I spoke to said the only solution was donor eggs and IVF. I eventually relented and did three rounds of IVF with horrendous side effects and still no pregnancy. That was enough.

I had given up, because giving up was the only way I found to cope after eighteen years of multiple treatments and constant failure to conceive.

I came to Gabriela (because my husband vehemently insisted) without hope but ready to try this one last time. After an incredibly thorough consultation, where we discussed all aspects of my health and fertility challenges, Gabriela suggested I might also have an issue with my thyroid. I hadn't been able to lose weight despite a healthy lifestyle and diet. She sent me for more tests, and we found out that Gabriela was right – I had a thyroid problem, along with many other minor factors we both needed to resolve. I did everything Gabriela asked, dutifully. Finally, there was some hope. Almost instantaneously I lost weight, normalised my cycle and felt so much better – as did my husband. I was irritated that after eighteen years on this rollercoaster, nobody had done all this.

It wasn't easy, and I had a lot of dark moments during that time. I also had a high-stress job. After feeling great for some months, suddenly one day I started feeling really unwell. I could barely get myself out of bed, I was nauseous and my asthma was bad. I spoke to Gabriela, and she ordered me to get a pregnancy test. I told her, 'Don't be ridiculous – I'm not pregnant! I probably just have the flu.' It couldn't possibly be true after almost twenty years of trying and failed IVF attempts. But I took two tests (in the middle of the night because I didn't want to get my husband's hopes up). One test came out positive and the other inconclusive. I went to the doctor first thing in the morning. She tested me, and sure enough it was positive. I still didn't believe it could be true.

At forty-six years old I had conceived – naturally, with my own eggs – and I delivered a beautiful, healthy baby girl.

A comprehensive testing protocol for thyroid function

If you're experiencing long-standing fertility problems and suspect thyroid involvement based on Tables 6.1 and 6.2, see your general medical practitioner, as further testing will be required to rule out thyroid disease.

Each patient's testing protocol is customised for each individual, however, as a general rule below is a big picture example of the questions we may pose biochemically when it comes to thyroid function. Although this is only one very small area of testing in the grand scheme of your fertility situation it is a very important one because scientific evidence is conclusive regarding the fact that imbalances arising here can categorically stop you (as a couple) from being able to get and stay pregnant.

The list of assays that follows can be ordered by the practitioner treating you. Piecing together and correlating your laboratory results with your clinical symptoms as well as your familial and previous medical history is an essential step towards beginning to understand your specific fertility situation and what else you may be required to do in order to transform your results.

The comprehensive thyroid testing protocol I use in my practice is as follows:

1. Thyrotropin-releasing hormone (TRH)

2. Thyroid function test or TSH. If TSH is higher than 2 mU/L, then include the following:

   a. fT4
   b. fT3
   c. rT3
   d. Thyroid antibodies:

      i. Thyroid peroxidase antibody (TPOAb)
      ii. Thyroglobulin antibody (TgAb)
      iii. Thyroid stimulating hormone receptor antibody (TRAb)

3. Vitamin D3

4. Iron study

5. Magnesium RBC

6. Selenium RBC

7. Copper/zinc ratio (serum copper and plasma zinc – tested together from same blood draw)

8. Iodine (twenty-four-hour urine)

9. Fasting insulin

10. Blood lipid panel (cholesterol, triglycerides)

11. AM fasting cortisol (start) or twenty-four-hour urinary cortisol excretion test or adrenal stress index (ASI) test

12. Oestradiol (E2) day two or three of menses (if female)

You'll mostly likely need help interpreting your results, and definitely do not attempt self-prescription in cases of imbalance because doing so will ensure you waste precious time on your fertility journey. Being proactive about your fertility, however, is the best way to fast-track your results.

Fertility Reset Prescription 8: Review your test results

The best way to ensure you have a holistic view of your current situation is to gather all of your previous test results, from every different practitioner you've seen over the years, and collate them into your own results folder.

Right now, it's important to ask yourself the following questions: Do you believe you've been properly investigated? What do you feel is missing to help you understand why you're struggling to conceive and take a healthy pregnancy to term? And most importantly, what else do you need to do to change your results?

Resources

Want to know how you can stop going around in circles on your fertility journey? Register for an obligation-free, complimentary fertility assessment and information session with our team.

Through the preparation required to participate in this session, you and your partner will come to understand with much greater clarity the obstacles you currently face and how to deal with them to optimise your chances of taking home a healthy baby. Register now: http://thefertile.me/NFBPInfoSession.

References

1   Morris, Z.S., et al., The answer is 17 years, what is the question: Understanding time lags in translational research. *Journal of the Royal Society of Medicine*, 2011. 104(12).

2   Bhat, A., et al. Infertility and perinatal loss: When the bough breaks. *Current Psychiatry Reports*, 2016. 18(3). www.ncbi.nlm.nih.gov/pmc/articles/PMC4896304

3   Frederiksen, Y., et al. Efficacy of psychosocial interventions for psychological and pregnancy outcomes in infertility women and men: A systematic review and meta-analysis. *BMJ Open*, 2015. 5(1). www.ncbi.nlm.nih.gov/pmc/articles/PMC4316425

4   Patel, A., et al. Role of mental health practitioner in infertility clinics: A review on past, present and future directions. *Journal of Human Reproductive Sciences*, 2018. 11(3). www.ncbi.nlm.nih.gov/pmc/articles/PMC6262662

5   Rooney, K.L., et al. The relationship between stress and infertility. *Dialogues in Clinical Neuroscience*, 2018. 20(1). www.ncbi.nlm.nih.gov/pubmed/29946210

6   Grunberg, P.H, et al. Infertility patients' need and preferences for online peer support. *Reproductive Biomedicine and Society Online*, 2018. 6. www.ncbi.nlm.nih.gov/pubmed/30547107

7   Wu, A.K., et al. Time costs of fertility care: The hidden hardship of building a family. *Fertility and Sterility*, 2013. 99(7). www.ncbi.nlm.nih.gov/pmc/articles/PMC3736984

8   Connolly, M.P., et al. The costs and consequences of assisted reproductive technology: An economic perspective. *Human Reproduction Update*, 2010. 16(6). www.ncbi.nlm.nih.gov/pubmed/20530804

9   Katz, P., et al. Costs of infertility treatment: Results from an 18-month prospective cohort study. *Fertility and Sterility*, 2011. 95(3). www.ncbi.nlm.nih.gov/pubmed/21130988

10   Dyer, S.J., et al. Catastrophic payment for assisted reproduction techniques with conventional ovarian stimulation in the public health sector of South Africa: Frequency and coping strategies. *Human Reproduction*, 2013. 28(10). www.ncbi.nlm.nih.gov/pubmed/23878180

11   Stuart, B., et al., Finding hope and healing when cure is not possible. *Mayo Clinic Proceedings*, 2019. 94(4).

12   Roudsari, R.L., et al., Looking at infertility through the lens of religion and spirituality: A review of the literature. *Human Fertility*, 2007. 10(3).

13   Zhao, T., et al., Meta-analysis of ART outcomes in women with different preconception TSH levels. *Reproductive Biology and Endocrinology: RB&E*, 2018. 16(1).

14   Zhang, Y., et al., Patients with subclinical hypothyroidism before 20 weeks of pregnancy have a higher risk of miscarriage: A systematic review and meta-analysis. *PLoS One*, 2017. 12(4)

15   Miko, E., et al., Characteristics of peripheral blood NK and NKT-like cells in euthyroid and subclinical hypothyroid women with thyroid autoimmunity experiencing reproductive failure. *Journal of Reproductive Immunology*, 2017. 124.

16   Seungdamrong, A., The impact and management of subclinical hypothyroidism for improving reproductive outcomes such as fertility and miscarriage. *Seminars in Reproductive Medicine*, 2016. 34(6).

17   Krassas, G.E., et al., Thyroid function and human reproductive health. *Endocrine Reviews*, 2010. 31(5).

18   La Vignera, S., et al., Thyroid dysfunction and semen quality. *International Journal of Immunopathology and Pharmacology*, 2018. 32.

19   La Vignera, S., et al., Impact of thyroid disease on testicular function. *Endocrine*, 2017. 58(3).

20   Wang, Y.-X., et al., Thyroid function, phthalate exposure and semen quality: Exploring associations and mediation effects in reproductive-aged men. *Environment International*, 2018. 116.

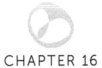

CHAPTER 16

Prescription 9:
Your Fertility Redefined With
The F.E.R.T.I.L.E. Method®

'Until you make the unconscious conscious,
it will direct your life and you will call it fate.'

Carl Jung

As humans, we desire, hope, wish, struggle, suffer and despair because, deep down, what we really want (and expect, to a lesser or greater degree) is to live in a transcendent state of perfection. Unfortunately, in this world, that place is only real in our fantastic imaginations. If you've ever thought, even for the slightest of moments, 'When I have X, then I'll be happy,' you know the place I mean – the place where all our desires and wishes show up exactly the way we want them and to which we compare and contrast everything in our lives. Our greatest disappointment is that the imagined version never seems to roll around the way we hoped it would. We want to forget that being human is being imperfect and that what this really means is that we don't simply get to stop working on ourselves. We will never be done and it will never be perfect. The sooner we accept this truth – fully and deeply, the sooner we can experience a different state of being.

Because let's be honest, no human exists whom has never thought, after much exertion (physical, mental, emotional, spiritual, you name it), 'I'm so glad I never have to do that again.' And really with due cause because when it comes to our physical and emotional maintenance (let alone progress) there hasn't ever been anything we could only just do once and it be done forever.

This is true for the basics of life like hygiene, eating, breathing, you name it. But somehow it feels equally true when applied to those things that sharply confront us and that eventually make us grow. It seems that especially, and somehow even more so, for the things that feel the hardest, we are constantly needing to review our life lessons that show up in different ways. It's as if a little time passes and – in need of some extra reminding of the previous learnings, further conditioning, or as some test of resolve to create real and lasting change – we are challenged, yet again, with some new situation (sometimes seemingly much harsher than the one before). I've lost count of how often my patients, in the depths of despair, turn their focus to 'why?' and 'why me?'.

It's easy to think that the circumstance is to blame – because 'surely, I've handled that already?' But the challenge is never the circumstance itself. What gets us in trouble in life is our perception of the situations we find ourselves in – the thought that it *should* just get easier to maintain the status quo of what we've already achieved. Another little thought may even rear its head: 'Surely I should be able to be, do, have everything I want from within, right here, in the cosiness of my comfort zone.'

Our angst is almost always a result of the internal rebellion against the contrast of what *is* versus what we would *rather* it be. We deeply desire *easy*. And when we're presented with something that's more challenging, difficult and heart-wrenching than we had imagined, we, more or less violently, dissent. Especially because other people, so much 'less deserving' just have it 'so easy'. (I've heard this thousands of times from patients over the years. You are not alone.)

I don't know about you specifically, but I could hazard a guess that your dissatisfaction regarding how things are on your fertility journey is fairly similar to that of my patients. For the most part, they struggle with some variation on the theme of 'my situation is harder, taking longer and costing more than I expected', even when they do their best to set realistic expectations.

What I've learned through observation over the years is that it's this mismatch of reality and expectation that makes most people despair. The truth is, we don't really want to work so much harder than we expected we'd have to in order to get what we want in life, especially when we have no iron-clad guarantee of attaining the result we strive towards – in every area.

What if fertility could be viewed as a metaphor to help us face what we'd rather dismiss in other areas of our lives?

Make a conscious choice

Some people will disagree and say, 'I'm happy to work hard for what I want.' And yes, we all are – as long as there's more pain in staying where we are than there is in making change. Beyond that is the point where all willingness wanes. Unless we can keep our eye on a higher purpose or objective, we end up making all sorts of excuses as to why we don't really need to stretch past our comfort zone.

It's perfectly fine to choose to be happy with what you have and decide you no longer want what you once did because the physical and emotional price is higher than you're willing to pay. But this decision must be a conscious one. It needs to come from a place of strong personal ownership, otherwise it's easy to fall into the trap of saying you didn't have or weren't enough to create what you wanted. We succumb to the role of the victim. This story is easy to tell ourselves. We make these sorts of excuses for our (sub- and unconscious) choices all the time. We say we don't have the money when the truth is we don't want to give up our nightly TV binge for a part-time job, or night college to upgrade our skills so we can get a better job and make more money. Or we choose to spend what we have on material possessions and expensive holidays. Or we simply don't want to invest because we don't see the value or we are afraid of making the wrong decision. All of these things are fine, but they all constitute a *choice*. A couple I worked with sold their car to undergo fertility treatment because they valued this more.

Tell yourself the truth. Don't make up a story about what you *can* and *can't* do when in reality, it's about what you *will* and *won't* do. Either way, your decision is perfectly valid. You don't need to justify it to anyone else. But you must be honest with yourself.

Once you're clear on your position, it's important to communicate your position with this same clarity to your partner. They need to understand where you're coming from and what you want or don't want because they also have the right to choose what's best for them based on their truth.

Untangle yourself from the biggest trap of all on the fertility journey: the story where you're a victim of your circumstances. That story, as compelling as it can appear, is never true. And the people who buy into this story are often the people who end up nursing some of the deepest regret of their lives. You always have a choice. Even if your choice is thinking differently about what you have.

It's about action. It's about doing everything you can to take charge and change your results. You have to ask yourself 'Have I really come this far to only come this far?' The status quo has a purpose, and it can also serve, but is it enough to serve you?

Perception is everything

A simple shift in perspective can transform everything (for better or worse) at the speed of thought.

It was running that first helped me internalise the fact that nothing (truly) is as hard as I make it out to be in my mind. Unlike my dad and sister, I've always been an 'anti-runner' (heavy weights in an air-conditioned gym are much more my thing – crazy, I know). For a long time, I thought there was something fundamentally wrong with my character because I lacked the willingness or grittiness (or both) to become a runner. But one day, I realised that I simply found the mental challenge of leg-pressing 200-plus kilos a whole lot more exciting than 'running from nothing' (my perception of the exercise).

In truth, I didn't value running. I had no desire to pursue it except to 'fit in' with my loved ones. Therefore, I couldn't grab on to any positive, motivating or inspiring associations to be able to really sustain it in the long term (because I hadn't bothered to create any – see Prescriptions 4 and 6).

Before realising all this, I really did work to get better at this running thing. I joined running clubs and did boot camps focused around running. And I went from dismally terrible at running to competent. To me, that was as much as I needed to feel that the challenge before me was conquered.

But before I got the lesson and the true blessing from the whole experience, I absolutely despised the days my trainer would make me run those damn uninterrupted five kilometres. And my complete and utter undoing would come on the days my trainer would say, 'OK, today you're going to run five kilometres. You'll smash it.' Then we'd reach the target and he'd say, 'Actually, we're doing another ten kilometres now.' Oh. My. Goodness.

You see, I would totally mentally prepare myself for five kilometres. I would prime my expectation of pain and discomfort and emotional suffering for that precise number of kilometres. I would store just enough resilience to take me through one lot of that pain, not three. Had it been an equivalent life circumstance, I likely would have ended up sobbing. It felt completely overwhelming. Looking back now (from the comfort of my office chair), excessively dramatic, really. But a good analogy.

Because what I gained from this experience, which seemed like Mount Everest in its enormity at the time, was a deep and utterly profound life lesson. The suffering didn't come from the experience or the situation itself. After I had a few goes at it, the challenge was by no means insurmountable. The depth of my suffering came only from my *unmet expectation* of how things should have been. The suffering was clearly optional, and only I could have chosen differently.

If my trainer had said, 'Right, today we're running fifteen kilometres', and then when I got to five, ten or even fourteen, he'd said, 'Actually, you're good, you've done enough, *X* was the real target – I just wanted to see if you'd go for it', I would have been ecstatic. Depending on how psyched up I was, I might have even chosen to finish the challenge. Regardless, I would have rejoiced in how (seemingly) easy and great the whole thing was.

Rationally, when the 'bad' running experience was over, I could admit to myself that things weren't as tragic as I'd made them out to be in my head. Let's be honest, though: most people aren't at their most rational amid great perceived distress. When I finally realised that how I reacted in this area of my life spilled over and coloured all other areas, it gave me a fresh, new perspective. I realised only I was responsible for getting caught up in the drama I continued to perpetuate, and only I could change it. Up until that point, I didn't know what I didn't know. I thought my unhappiness had been 'given to me' by this unpleasant experience. Instead, it had been up to me all along.

And with this understanding, I began to see that standard treatment was simply not good enough to help couples deal with the real problems causing their symptoms (including the lack of baby) – we needed to dig deeper. Much deeper.

It was from this place that I began shaping the treatment we have now successfully delivered for many years in my clinic. And the benefits our patients began experiencing through the application of the F.E.R.T.I.L.E. Method® throughout their journey with us quickly encompassed every aspect of their lives – not just their fertility and reproductive outcomes.

How the F.E.R.T.I.L.E. Method® came to be

The approach that now serves as my team's treatment compass emerged (and is constantly refined) as a result of our combined experience and observation of the couples we treat, but it's also based on the latest findings in human psychology and behaviour. Since we specialise in difficult and complex cases, a fully customised and individualised process based on a solid and proven framework is essential to optimise results.

I saw a need to formalise this approach to ensure its consistent delivery within my practice and as a result, the F.E.R.T.I.L.E. Method® was born.

The critical importance of a solid framework was first brought to my attention by American surgeon, public health researcher and Harvard professor Atul Gawande, author of *The Checklist Manifesto*.[1] He borrowed wisdom from the aviation industry and made a great case for why surgery (or any important endeavour) should never begin or end without a comprehensive checklist – checked off, no matter how simple the task might seem. He also provided a great illustration (in words, scientific results and the cost in numbers and lives) of how much can go wrong when the checklist and its simple, yet remarkable concept are ignored.

I took this idea and applied it to every aspect of what a couple and my team need to consider in terms of optimising fertility, from beginning to baby (and beyond). Consequently, the F.E.R.T.I.L.E. Method® has become the effective step-by-step process that powers the incredible results we are able to help our patients achieve on the Natural Fertility Breakthrough Program™.

This methodology is also the driving force behind our educational efforts, which has now seen The Fertility Challenge™ be able to provide over 100,000 couples in more than 100 countries with effective education to take charge of their health and fertility.

The truth is our babies are the cherries on top, but the education and inspiration that leads to the transformation of thousands of lives is truly the reason I keep showing up after all these years, and the reason why I'm inspired to do even more.

I think it's fair to say that given all of my life and professional experiences, I have developed a deep, unwavering faith in effective systems and processes. I know that if I'm not where I want to be in any area of my life, I need to examine my system and my process. Once I'm satisfied that the system is effective and it has got me facing in the right direction, it's a matter of keeping at it, even when I'm 'over it' and bored with doing what it takes. It then all becomes about process. Because I know that little by little, I'm getting my result. The reason it's important to set your mind to doing whatever it takes for as long as it takes is that getting bored with doing what it takes happens on the journey, infinitely sooner than results. However, at the first whiff of boredom is where most people will quit. Not the people who achieve above-average results, of course, but typically the people without a solid strategy and adequate accountability in place.

It isn't always easy to keep going until, not if, you get your results. I'll be the first to admit this. But choosing to develop this 'keep going' attitude has served my patients and I well, and it's the solid foundation upon which the repeatable success of the F.E.R.T.I.L.E. Method® rests.

Now is the time to be happy

'Progress is impossible without change, and those who cannot change their minds cannot change anything.'

George Bernard Shaw

Over the decades, my patients have taught me that when a couple wrestles for years with infertility and recurrent miscarriage, typically much more than a baby is required to overcome the aftermath of this hardship. There is often deep trauma associated with such a struggle, which standard therapy acknowledges but does little to effectively address. This is why I believe in working through whatever is necessary to enable you to thrive and live your best life now while working towards your dream of parenthood. You must also learn to see what is wonderful about where you stand right now, because you won't ever be happy 'when' if you can't be happy 'now' – irrespective of the challenges you currently face.

Nothing and no one outside of you can give you happiness. Not even a child. It's not their responsibility to make you happy. It's yours. And putting your best, healthiest and most fulfilled life on hold until something outside of you shows up (as wonderful as babies are) means you're wishing away the goodness already in your life.

Babies are not dolls. They are people, with their own wants, wishes and desires. And if their actions don't match your expectations, you might still be unhappy if you don't learn what it takes to be happy now. In fact, as I write this, the universe is providing me with a perfect example. I'm sitting in the food court of a busy shopping centre, and a few feet from me is a toddler throwing a tantrum – it's a good one, complete with lying on the floor and ear-piercing screeches. The mother is totally flustered and exasperated.

Let's say you focus on how perfect your life will be when you're finally pregnant and finally have a baby. And then your child, like mine, doesn't sleep for more than an hour and twenty minutes (most often, though, no more than twenty minutes) throughout the day or night for the first eight months of his life. Also, he *never* lets you put him down anywhere. You get two or three thirty-minute stretches of sleep a night for months on end. In this case, you must be able to draw on a different kind of strength to 'get through'. And when will you develop it, if not now?

Having clarity about what you want to create is vital. You must be unwavering on the 'what' but flexible on the 'how'. And developing the resilience and strength of mind that ends up making everything else possible is the only way to live your best life now. It will never be easier. You will just have to become even more resourceful.

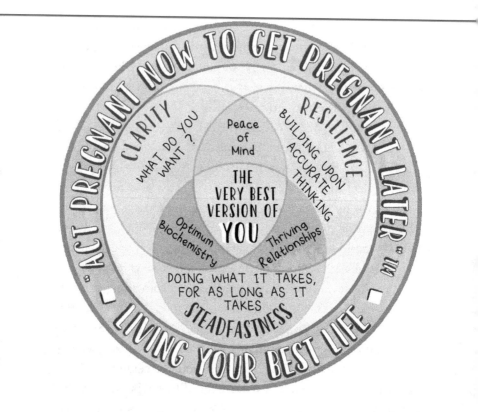

My patients have shown me that from this place of strength, you're much more likely to make the choices necessary to support you and your partner in creating your dream. This is why I developed the F.E.R.T.I.L.E. Method® with these tenets (clarity, steadfastness and resilience) in the forefront of my mind.

A healthy and well-balanced individual contributes to better relationships and experiences a greater quality of life in the process of creating better fertility outcomes. Therefore, in the simplest visual terms, the F.E.R.T.I.L.E. Method® has one aim: to help you create the best version of you. From there, everything else flows.

Putting the F.E.R.T.I.L.E. Method® into practice

While working with thousands of patients on every continent, my team and I identified three key problems all couples experience at some point on their journey through fertility difficulties. You may already have personal experience with them.

- **Problem #1** – They feel the ticking of their biological clock is deafening and are stumped as to *why* they aren't getting pregnant

- **Problem #2** – They are heartbroken by their lack of tangible results and can't shake off the unpleasantness of feeling like they've tried everything and nothing has worked

- **Problem #3** – They're tired of putting their life on hold and overwhelmed by all the contradictory advice they've received

Seeing and experiencing this suffering with my patients, I wanted to alleviate it. I passionately wanted to help people on this journey, to show them how to take advantage of the tools and strategies available to them. I'd always felt the solutions for couples experiencing fertility difficulties needed to be reimagined to deliver more than a healthy baby. This was the place I wanted to start from.

Now, the results speak for themselves.

The people who get the best results through implementing our methodology are ready to do what it takes, with our help. Our patients are those who are willing to be coachable through a proven process. All the while willing to dig deep to find their strength. They are not archetypically the 'lucky' ones but they sure rise from the ashes.

I'll be honest – the results I've seen over the years and continue to experience creating with our patients still surprise me. Our patients are not numbers on some statistical curve. In fact, they typically behave in ways that are quite opposite to those that make the statistical curves possible. For this and many other reasons, I'm a huge proponent of 'getting in there and doing the work'. Because as so many of my patients have said to me over the years, and their babies' lives categorically prove – the process can work, if you do.

MIRACLE MOMENTS

• WE DID EVERYTHING
GABRIELA TOLD US TO DO •
AMANDA AND ALEX

The heartbreak of recurrent miscarriage was really taking its toll on me and my husband, Alex. I had lost triplets due to a cervical issue, and I can't even begin to describe what that felt like. With another round of IVF I managed to conceive, but I miscarried again. We were really struggling to understand what was going wrong. I had a really hard time processing why I couldn't have a child.

We decided to do IVF again, and at the end of yet another failed cycle, we knew we needed to do something different. I spent hours researching online and finally found Gabriela and called to make an appointment. After an extensive assessment with Gabriela and her team, we decided to apply for the Natural Fertility Breakthrough Program™. Fortunately, we eventually got a place and were able to get started.

Gabriela showed me the right approach to take for my specific problem. She taught me how to heal my body, and how to make it healthy and strong. We dedicated ourselves to the program, day in, day out. We chose to do it. We did everything Gabriela asked us to do. We were completely single-minded about it. If Gabriela said we should do it, we did it with determination and to the best of our abilities.

We were facing factors that made IVF our best option so with the team's support we embarked on our next cycle. My egg quality was so healthy compared to three years previously when this whole journey had started, and I needed minimal drugs because my body was so healthy. I got pregnant on the first round. I didn't believe we could have a baby so quickly after all we'd been through. But we did it together.

My husband and I bonded through this process, through our efforts together. Nothing can describe the feeling of having a baby when you think for so long that you'll never have one. We had our daughter, Abby, and when she was three years of age, and after revisiting the program, I gave birth to our twin girls, Livvy and Maddie.

Focus throughout the process is absolutely necessary. And what we also know from our patients' experiences over the years is that doing what it takes, consistently, and ideally as a couple delivers even better results. On average our patients take home babies between twelve to thirty-six months from beginning the process (taking into account a nine-month pregnancy). This period includes three highly personalised and carefully constructed treatment stages: preconception preparation, conception attempts, and pregnancy and postnatal care.

Each couple works with several specialist clinicians (each focused on their own area of expertise) who appropriately stage each step in our treatment process for the patients we're privileged to serve. I have structured things in this way because in my opinion, a truly effective, holistic protocol cannot possibly be delivered by one person – no matter how good they are at what they do. From seeing our highly skilled team in action over the years, I have also come to believe that when great minds combine in the pursuit of a complete solution for a patient's case – as a group, we are sharper, infinitely faster and more effective than one clinician who tries to tackle a highly complex and multifactorial problem on their own. Therefore, I leverage my team's expertise for the benefit of our patients in everything we do. We're here to help our patients create their dream – no matter how difficult it may have been in the past. I'm unphased by the difficulty of the task. I care about results.

We accept patients into our program based on certain criteria because over the years, I've seen that what we do works best for a particular type of person: someone who intrinsically knows that they're looking for something very specific. Let me explain.

We work with couples who have been trying to conceive or take home a healthy baby for over two years; or who have experienced miscarriages; or who have three or more minor factors (see 'The Minor Things To Major In' in Part 1) getting in their way. The couples we work with want to leave nothing to chance and no stone unturned. Our patients want more, and they're ready to be guided and to work for it.

To be a good fit for our treatment, patients must be willing to invest the time, the energy, the effort and the money, but most importantly, they must be fully committed to working through a proven process. They must be coachable. We will always clarify and provide evidence of everything we recommend, but at some point people just have to be willing to get on with it and do what it takes.

Everything we ask our patients to do we've done ourselves. None of it is superhuman, but none of it is up for debate – because breakthroughs are not a given. Breakthroughs must be created, and they certainly aren't created by magic. I'll be honest: our style is more Spartan than spa treatment. I have high standards and expectations for myself, and I have the same expectations for my team and my patients.

You will need to answer more questions than you've ever been asked before. You may need to go through more tests and investigations (even if you feel you have already done all there is, I promise, it's likely you haven't scratched the surface of what is needed to have clear and definitive answers about your specific situation). All of these factors combined make up a huge part of the reason why we're able to get results for our patients, even after everything else has failed.

If anything I've just described doesn't resonate with you, that's perfectly fine – it simply means that you will still benefit greatly from everything I share in this book but working one-on-one with our clinic isn't for you. Our in-house service is for people whose 'inner knowing' says, 'Yes, this is what I'm looking for!' I want you to have everything in life you want and I have zero interest in convincing anyone that they should do our program. We are in our patients' lives for a long time – in many cases forever (we often keep in touch for years). And I think we will agree that life is simply too short to live out of alignment with one's choices. Our patients deeply connect with what is required to transform their results.

The F.E.R.T.I.L.E. Method® explained

Once resonance is established, we can take each step through the F.E.R.T.I.L.E. Method® together, from beginning to baby. Let's take a look at the steps.

F: Fact-find – Imagine that fertility is a 1,000-piece puzzle. But there's no box with a clear picture on the front, and the pieces are scattered in unknown places. A 'treasure hunt' is required (but most couples go through a wild goose chase). Hence, the first step of the F.E.R.T.I.L.E. Method® involves looking for and pulling together all the pieces required to give us an idea of what the image on the front of the box would look like (and how we may need to adjust it). With the help of expertly trained clinicians, couples are guided through a series of specific physical, emotional and biochemical assessments to discover some of the minor and major factors keeping them stuck. I'm unrelenting about constant improvement, so our protocols are always evolving and incorporating new directions in treatment as scientific evidence emerges.

E: Educate – Our patients and their babies are living proof that education, inspiration and consistent application (with high account-ability) gets results. I've also learned over many years that when people can't link their behaviour to a positive (or negative) outcome (which is hard to do in the day to day), or they are uneducated about why something matters in helping them achieve their results, nothing happens. Ultimately, simply knowing something and not applying it produces zero effect. In essence this lack of action translates into the very same outcome as not knowing that potentially transformational piece of information at all. Most people fail to modify their behaviour not because they don't want to create positive, lasting change but because they've never been taught an effective way to do so.

The people who are attracted to our clinic are not 'the masses'. Typically, they are high-functioning individuals and couples who want more for their lives and are stuck as to how to get it. When we first meet, they might be feeling down, but they don't envision themselves as victims of circumstances.

Our style of treatment resonates with people who will continue to get up, dust themselves off and resolve to create *choice* for themselves in their lives – even if at times they need to be assisted back onto their feet. Not everyone who goes through our treatment will end up with a baby. But every single person will know, categorically, what choices they can make along the journey (and beyond) while living their best life. They will never have to wonder if they did enough. They will know. There is huge freedom in that.

R: Recommend – Only after a comprehensive fact-find can we begin to make personalised recommendations for patients. Then, each couple receives evidence-based and customised recommendations regarding every one of their 11 Pillars of Fertility Foundations™. In the first instance, the aim is always a biological clean-up to remove obstacles to optimum health and fertility, 'Marie Kondo' style (the ultimate goal is joy).

T: Treat – This is the fourth step, not the first, for a reason. Many treatment providers begin their process with 'Here – take this and inject that' only to conduct further investigations later when things don't go to plan, claiming you have no time to waste. I agree you have no time to waste. But trying to address and optimise fertility in retrospect is like trying to pin the tail on the donkey while blindfolded. It's a questionable strategy, to say the least. We prefer to do the work to identify and collect the puzzle pieces first. We take great care to systematically remove the obstacles we already know of through our patients' (carefully elicited) self-reporting and incorporate the new findings we discover along the way, all the while carefully measuring and monitoring our patients' responses to treatment. If you have no time to waste on your fertility journey, don't waste it on not systematically implementing these steps. This is the most important work – the 20% of the effort that gives our patients 80% of their result and can make the difference between having a baby or not. Most couples apply themselves in the wrong way. They do 80% of the stuff that yields 20% of their result, and then understandably become exhausted by their efforts and arrive at that well-known place of 'I've tried everything and nothing has worked'.

There is always more that *can* be done. The question is, do you want to do it?

I: Incubate – As I've said, you can't hack biology. You have just as much control over how long it takes for the egg to mature (about eight months) and the sperm to form (a minimum of four months) as you do over the fact that a human pregnancy is nine months long, or that the sun rises and sets each day (unless you live really far north or south). Wanting to speed everything up will do only one thing – distract you from what you can actually influence to create your result. It's up to you to learn to mindfully let go of the need to control the uncontrollable. There is great power in that.

It might feel as if nothing is happening during the incubation process, but it's a critical step. Think of a seed just underneath the soil. As the plant prepares to poke through, there's much activity happening that you can't see. You may feel disheartened and want to give up on the process (the daily watering and feeding of 'the seed'). But giving up now will simply give you more of what you had before.

Steadfastly doing the work in pursuit of your dream and seeing its eventual accomplishment is so much more fulfilling than all the other possible alternatives combined.

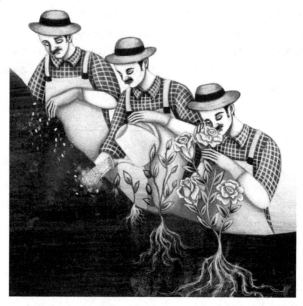

During this stage of the process, we continue to collect new puzzle pieces and adjust our prescriptions and treatment recommendations – each step getting us closer to the best version of you. Various members of our team are available for extra support here. The key at this stage is for the couple (or individual) not to lose sight of the goal and what's required to achieve it.

L: Liberate – This is the huge mindset piece of this journey, and a part of the process that happens concurrently with every other step. My aim is to help couples look at their situation from a completely different perspective and learn how to draw strength from their circumstances rather than dip into victim mentality. Our patients prove to me daily that living life is much more enjoyable from their centre of personal power and strength. This step requires willingness coupled with the right tools and strategies.

E: End result – The F.E.R.T.I.L.E. Method® wouldn't be complete without this step; this step is a cause for celebration. Irrespective of how a couple achieves their dream of parenthood while creating the best versions of themselves, most couples tell us at this stage how relieved and happy they feel about having given it their all for the sake of themselves and their future.

As mentioned, not every couple goes on to have a baby. Some choose to draw their line in the sand about what they won't do to create a baby. And as far as I'm concerned, this is perfect. People, as well as their wishes and desires, change along the path. Choice is freedom, and I couldn't want anything more for my patients.

Remember Tracey and Paul – after ten years of failed attempts and unsuccessful IVF treatments, they conceived after a short time on our fertility program and went on to have their happy and healthy baby, Tyler. Emma and Tom – after eight miscarriages, they now have four beautiful healthy children. And Megan and Josh – after extended infertility and the heartbreak of miscarriage, they went on to naturally conceive and deliver a healthy set of male triplets and a couple of years later a healthy baby girl. These results happened because these couples took charge of their health and fertility and consistently applied what we teach. Perfection is overrated, but you can do what it takes for as long as it takes, steadfastly, utilising the best strategies possible.

These results don't just magically or 'accidentally' occur. Our results happen by design. Focus, effort and determination are required for any couple who wishes to transform their results.

There are things on the fertility journey that you and your partner, and only you and your partner can do. If you really want to stack the odds in your favour, you must take charge.

References

1   Gwandi, A., *The Checklist Manifesto: How to Get Things Right*. 2011, New York: Henry Holt and Company.

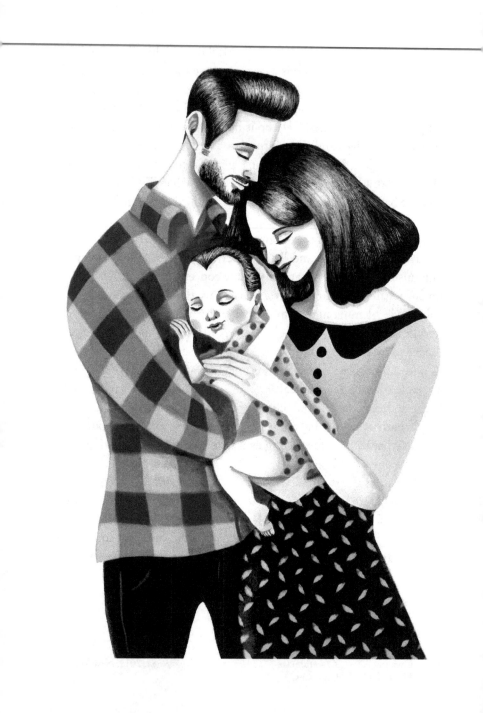

PART 3

YOU'VE GOT THIS.
AND I'VE GOT YOU.

'Until one is committed there is hesitancy,
the chance to drawback, always ineffectiveness.'

William Hutchison Murray

I once heard that we overestimate what we can achieve in one year
and completely underestimate we can do in a decade. For some
areas of life, this may be very true. However, when infertility
and miscarriage mark the journey to parenthood with such major
ups and downs, which end up spanning across multiple years or
even decades, it's easy to feel like nothing is being accomplished –
especially as the physical and emotional costs of the whole situation
continue to mount.

It doesn't take too long on this journey for couples to withdraw
into the fears and disappointments they've experienced. Fearing
they will never have their result, and in an effort to have some
aspect of control over their journey, without knowing who they can
trust, they start to obsess about every little thing they read or hear
about that could help them have a baby. As a result, they end up
piling on more 'stuff' to their to-do lists, except that unfortunately
because they can only see one side of the whole equation, it ends
up being mostly inconsequential (the 80% of the effort that only
delivers 20% of the result). And this is sadly how most couples

who don't experience immediate success on this journey become overwhelmed, exhausted and bitterly disappointed – ultimately because they have committed to the wrong strategy.

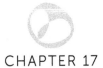

CHAPTER 17

Create Your Own
Fertility Breakthrough

T he biggest trap couples I speak to fall into is thinking they can turn their fertility journey into a 'do-it-yourself' project. And then there are the couples who still have a solid chance of taking home a healthy baby if they do the work but instead of taking immediate, decisive action decide on some alternate route – only to come back to me three years later and say, 'Now I'm ready to get started.' When it comes to fertility, three years, heck, three months, is a long time.

Remember, the egg takes about eight months to fully mature. We start seeing physiological changes upon implementing new strategies at about six months, meaning that if you delay starting by three months, we are already a minimum of nine months away from the desired improvements. A six-month delay means we're talking about a minimum twelve months to begin seeing results, and that's assuming conception happens immediately. Some people simply don't have that amount of time to simply waste on their journey. Add another nine months (gestation) and we're twenty-one months from when you first became aware that there was more you could do. And if you'd like to have more than one child, time is even more precious.

Women tend to grasp this concept sooner because we're well aware that our fertility is decidedly finite. Men, on the other hand, often underestimate this fact and take a more casual approach to how much extra assistance is necessary to overcome the difficulties they are facing. An overly relaxed approach (as a couple) can have an extremely detrimental effect on your chances of taking home a healthy baby.

I want to make something clear – if any of what I've just said applies to you (and/or your partner), you need to take decisive action now, in whatever way feels right for you. Because it could make the difference between you creating your dream of parenthood or not.

• TIME IS OF THE ESSENCE •

Definitive action is required now, not later, if you:

- Have been trying to conceive for over two years (and you're under thirty); or for as little as three months after thereafter if either partner is dealing with one or more obstacles to optimum fertility

- Have experienced at least one miscarriage or chemical pregnancy

- Have more than one known minor factor (or obstacle to optimum health and fertility) – see 'The Minor Things To Major In' in Part 1

- Have undergone fertility treatment, such as ovulation-stimulation drugs, IUI or IVF/ICSI, that's failed

- Lead a healthy lifestyle and are generally quite health conscious but are still not pregnant after more than three appropriately timed conception attempts

Time is of the essence, so you must ensure you're using it appropriately, with an effective and proven strategy in place.

Whatever you do, don't underestimate the enormity of this task. I say this not to alarm you, but to put things into context. What you've come to believe about your chances of conception might be only a small piece of the puzzle you need to assemble, against the clock. I want you to know it's possible. But you need to act – now.

• TAKE A BREATH •

Ask yourself, 'What do I really want?' Are you ready to take charge and make your own luck? Reach out for the extra help you need and begin.

Start counting the real costs

'Everything comes at a cost.
Just what are you willing to pay for it?'

Serena Williams

Prevention is always cheaper than cure. But infertility prevention isn't exactly straightforward. For one, fertility isn't discussed as an educational topic when it matters most: the teenage years. If you knew then what you know now, your conversations, let alone your actions, would likely have been much different.

Teenagers are educated on the 'horrors' of teen pregnancy and how easily an unwanted pregnancy can happen. They're taught the importance of using contraception. But they're given very little, if any, information on how to optimise their bodies in a proactive way for when, years later, fertility is desired.

Teens aren't taught about the importance of dietary and lifestyle choices that safeguard future fertility,[1,2,3] or the devastating impact of sexually transmitted infections, specifically on fertility and chances of conception.[4,5,6,7] To say nothing of what endocrine disruptors are, where they're found, and the long-term impact they have on a couple's fertility.[8,9]

But it's very much in those teen years that education about infertility prevention is essential. This public health concern cannot continue to be neglected. In 'sex ed' classes, boys and girls are never taught that a woman has a twelve- to twenty-four-hour chance of getting pregnant in any given month because that's the lifespan of the egg – at her most fertile, a woman has a (maximum) 20% chance of conceiving in any given cycle.[10,11]

I believe teenagers should be educated about their reproductive cycles in a less biased way. Girls should be encouraged to track their reproductive cycles and understand how their bodies work so they're acutely aware of when they're actually fertile and when they're not – so, in due course, they know when to double their efforts with contraception, abstain from unprotected intercourse or time conception attempts to optimise their chances of conceiving. And, like my patients, they should also be encouraged to educate their partners on these matters, so men are equally aware of the realities of the female reproductive cycle (way before the pressures, challenges and struggles of infertility may arise).

Instead, our society is taught to medicate. We're taught to take a pill for when we don't want to conceive and one for when we do, without so much as a second thought about the long-term effects of our actions. Teenagers become the infertility patients of the future as the system continues to feed them with more medication than education. And as this cycle perpetuates itself, infertility rates slowly but steadily increase, along with corporate profits, while you remain unaware, or strategically made to forget, that you have a choice.

When couples visit their general practitioner for their allotted seven-minute consultation for help trying to conceive, they aren't asked any questions about lifestyle, nor are they given any counsel, guidance or education on effective ways to improve their fertility outcomes. Instead, they're given a referral to IVF/ICSI to be told when they should report for the start of a cycle or simply that they need donor egg or donor embryo. At which point most people panic and jump into the ever-growing assisted-reproduction funnel. From there, they begin the injections, the monitoring appointments and the stress and anticipation that comes with each day of that cycle, culminating at the end with that anticipated, yet dreaded, phone call from the clinic to report on the result of it all. And when the outcome is a negative pregnancy test, patients are often just told it's a 'numbers game' and without further ado, the next cycle is scheduled. And so it continues.

Some couples eventually conceive this way. However, most (which is more than 65%, given that the average IVF clinic's success rate is approximately 20% to 30%) continue spiralling down into despair and exhaustion (physical, emotional and financial) until some eventually run out of time all together.[12]

All the while, the costs to the individual (physical and emotional), as well as the drain that constantly trying to get pregnant places on finances, the relationship and one's own self-esteem, continue on unaddressed (sometimes for years) – as the couple's biological clock rushes through countdown mode.

And this pattern continues in our society despite mounting scientific evidence clearly showing that optimising fertility by addressing obstacles to health before a conception attempt halves the number of cycles required to take home a baby via IVF – and potentially rendering it completely unnecessary.[13,14,15,16,17,18,19] This crucial education isn't making it through to patients via mainstream media or the very clinics that provide the service.

At some point, a high percentage of couples hit rock bottom. The pain of their unattained dreams and the realisation of their depleted finances signal the first big stop sign on their fertility journey.

It doesn't have to be this way.

Upon some reflection, many couples go back for more of the same. But a few unique individuals realise the answer lies not in more of the same but in taking a much more holistic approach. These couples are ready to ask more questions, and deeper questions. They realise the transformation must begin from the inside out. They begin to consider all the costs.

It's true that we'll always find money to invest in what we value most, but it's important to consider the aggregate impact of your investments in every area of your life and what each investment gets you and others it touches in the long term. In other words, whatever path you choose, you need to ask yourself: 'Is it good for me?' 'Is it good for my prospective child?' and 'Is it good for the planet I'll eventually leave behind?'

Your reasons for doing or not doing something will always be valid to you in the moment but consider this litmus test, which I like to use in my life: ask yourself, 'How will this choice feel when I'm ninety, sitting on my porch in my rocking chair?' The one thing I know my patients will never regret is doing their best and giving it their all in a way that respects them and those who are affected by their decisions.

Finally, here's something else to keep in mind: it's easy to see the mounting expenses of optimising fertility and forget to acknowledge the lifetime cost of having a child. The truth is, if you think getting pregnant is too expensive, know that providing for a child until the age of eighteen is a bill estimated at upwards of $1,000,000.[20] And this sum can end up being much more in different parts of the world due to escalating costs of education and living. As well, children are staying at home longer – until, on average, twenty-four years of age.[21,22] A hefty investment indeed. Yet, for some couples struggling to conceive, one that must begin before conception – if the dream of a baby is ever to be realised.

• TAKE A BREATH •

Every decision attracts a cost. But the real question you need to ask yourself is, 'What will it cost me in the future – physically, emotionally, financially, spiritually, in terms of relationships, etc – to delay doing everything I can now?'

So, before rushing into any incomplete strategy, thinking it's your only solution, take charge of creating your own fertility breakthrough (follow the process outlined in this book or participate in one of my other programs). Work to address the known obstacles to your optimum health and fertility, and work to uncover and resolve as many others as can be found through in-depth investigations in the most holistic, methodical and systematic way possible to ensure nothing is left to chance.

> 'Whatever you think you can do or believe you can do, begin it. Action has magic, grace and power in it.'
>
> Wolfgang von Goethe

You're not alone – fertility is a team sport

Keep the faith, do what it takes, and enjoy the ride.

Some couples fail to align with what's required from each other to overcome infertility and miscarriage. They fail to get educated and realise too late that taking home a healthy baby is dependent on the participation of two fully committed parties. Riding a tandem bicycle is fun, but only if your partner is willing to pedal as much as you – especially when most of the way might be uphill. Otherwise, the fun turns to blame. And in the case of the fertility journey, blame is coupled with feelings of loneliness, despair and disappointment when the going gets tough.

When it comes to fertility, it doesn't matter whose 'fault' it is. In fact, I never, ever look at minor-factor distribution in a couple in this way. The job is to figure out what we need to do to optimise your fertility as a couple, as your very own team.

Typically, if you're told that the egg-quality score on your team is low, you're not told that in order to have the best possible chance of taking home a healthy baby, the sperm needs to be of the highest quality. Biologically speaking, it's the egg's responsibility to address and optimise the genetic imperfections not routinely seen under the microscope (yet present) within the sperm. So, if the egg is struggling, the 'less work' it has to do in terms of promoting the sperm's viability, the more likely each partner's input is to contribute to the creation of a viable embryo. This ultimate creation can only happen as a result of effective teamwork. Even if you opt for donor egg, donor sperm or donor embryo, there's no escaping doing the preparatory work. You need to neutralise the effects of the minor or major obstacles. And you've got to question the motives of anyone who tells you otherwise.

Don't think that you're off the hook just because your blood tests came back fine, or your semen analysis was 'above average'. If you want to give yourself the best possible chance of revolutionising your results, both prospective parents must commit to this process for themselves and together, to really create that much-needed transformation in biochemistry

If you're in a happy, loving and connected relationship and would like to be in one for a long time, understand that helping your partner reach their dream is the ultimate result in itself. That's what creates happy and strong marriages. Being together as a team, doing what it takes, is crucial to get the results that you're looking for.

I'm originally from Brazil and have been to the Amazon several times. The last time I went, I took my husband with me for the first time. We stayed in a magnificent place, 100 kilometres into the Amazon jungle. One morning, we canoed on the Amazon River and waited for the sun to come up. Where we were, the river was so wide all we could see was the water and the horizon. Slowly, incredible rays of pinks, oranges, yellows and blues appeared. It was the most magnificent sight of my whole life, and I got to experience it with my husband, my partner, my love.

As I explained that wondrous sunrise, you probably got the gist of my experience. But you didn't get the full experience. You would have had to be there yourself to see it and experience it for yourself. Creating your fertility breakthrough works the same way. You both have to be there, to do the work, to get the aha moments. If you're not sharing things with your partner, they'll miss out on understanding them for themselves.

Fertility, like many other things in life, isn't fifty-fifty in the sense that you bring your 50% and your partner brings their 50%. No, both parties must bring their 100%. In this equation, if you're both bringing only 50%, you'll both have only a quarter of a whole. This isn't psychology. It's mathematics.

For years now, I've seen how important it is for couples to work on overcoming infertility together – to better their health and their ability to work well together as a team before a baby enters the picture. In doing so, they build the solid family foundation so important for raising a healthy and well-adjusted child. This is why family foundations is one of the very important 11 Pillars of Fertility Foundations™, as well as why the Natural Fertility Breakthrough Program™ places emphasis on relationship and personal development work. This focus ensures our patients have the tools and skills to create a healthy relationship and a happy family living their best life in preparation to welcome their baby in the future.

• TAKE A BREATH •

Are you working together as a team? How else can you support each other? What can you do today to educate and inspire your partner into action? It's not enough to have either education or inspiration – to make this work, you need both.

Your best imperfect self is all that's required

'Most things don't work out as expected, but what happens instead often turns out to be the good stuff.'

Dame Judi Dench

By now you know that I believe perfection is highly overrated. Falling is inevitable. What I want to know is how many times you'll get back up. Getting up for the umpteenth time is a choice – and one that only you can make.

Overcoming infertility and recurrent miscarriage is a journey, even though it feels like a destination. Sometimes you'll make a wrong turn. And sometimes things out of your control will go wrong, leaving you with nothing but necessary course correction. It's important to expect this from the outset and resolve that you will do whatever it takes – not just when it's easy and you have all the excitement of a new journey behind your sails, but when it counts the most in those dark moments when all you have to rely upon is the faith that you're facing in the right direction. You must continue, steadfastly, moving forward in the direction of the dream you want to create.

Most couples struggling through long-term infertility and recurrent miscarriage start to focus on the wrong things, such as why it's taking so long for their early efforts to yield fruit. Instead, you need to concentrate on tending the soil and watering and feeding the seed. You need to measure and celebrate (most importantly celebrate) 'little by little' progress.

Focusing on your why and your outcome is important but if you are only focused on your outcome, without enjoyment and appreciation for what you have already created and achieved, it is so easy (especially when things are difficult) to become discouraged and give up – often just before that little green blade pushes through to the surface.

This is why you commit and decide in advance that you will do whatever it takes to get your result – whatever that looks like. As mentioned before, you must absolutely draw a line, but don't quit mid-strategy. Your dream is too important to make decisions during a time of heightened and volatile emotions. You need your wits about you and you need to apply your best thinking so you can be part of your solution.

My patients categorically prove that overcoming infertility and recurrent miscarriage when other treatments have failed is as much about grit as it is about leveraging the right strategy. Fine tuning and adjustment must always be part of a comprehensive plan, but jumping around from one strategy to another will never get you the results you want.

There's no point wishing things were different. You need to commit to solid strategy and follow it through until completion. Just know and accept that yes, you'll need to dig in deeper and do even more. (Remember the Heroin Addict Syndrome story we mentioned earlier?) We wouldn't be here having this conversation otherwise. But the end and its result you determine.

And remember, this isn't about fairness. If your unhealthy sister, neighbour or whoever got pregnant 'accidentally', you need to accept that you're on a different journey. And then get to work. Either that or you must decide that you're OK with not having a baby. And then go make your life the masterpiece you want it to be in a different way. Flexibility is often required on this path, and sometimes even regarding how you'll become a parent (there could very well be a need to consider strategies such as surrogacy, donor egg/sperm, etc).

One of my patients said it best: 'My biggest takeaway from working with you is that I'm not a victim of infertility. As a couple, we previously made choices that have, most likely, contributed to our infertility. Although I can't change that, I can make better choices now that will benefit my health and happiness, and support me towards my objective of having a healthy baby. Through this journey, my husband and I have realised that while having a healthy baby is a goal of ours, being healthy, happy and grateful for all we already have and for each other is our main goal. I'm so grateful for this experience.'

• TAKE A BREATH •

Stop beating yourself up. Educate yourself and simply do your best. If you still feel a baby is part of your destiny, then be ready to do the work. In the end, everything is work. Crying about what you don't have is just as much work as making better choices for yourself – persistently and consistently. The latter has the potential to make your dreams come true. What will you choose?

What if it never happens?

'Nothing gets transformed in your life until
your mind is transformed.'

Ifeanyi Enoch Onuoha

We find ourselves in a unique time in history where, given enough willingness, effort and money, most couples can create and fulfil their dream of parenthood. Only you can draw your 'line in the sand'.

So many patients have told me that when their baby enters their family, it doesn't matter by what means they arrived. Not every method of having a baby fits with every couple's hopes, dreams, desires and beliefs, though – and it's necessary to acknowledge this at every stage along the way. It was only as late as 1978 that IVF made its debut; the first donor egg procedure was still five years away, and the first donor embryo cycle was only deemed ethical and feasible in 1986. These procedures didn't become mainstream until much later, and their availability was restricted to geographical pockets (mainly the United States).[23,24] We've come a long way in terms of reproductive treatment feasibility, accessibility and choice. When I first started supporting couples who wanted to overcome infertility and miscarriage (in Australia circa 2001), no amount of willingness, effort and money was enough for most couples struggling to take home a healthy baby. Still, there's a long way to go in terms of standardising effective, holistic fertility care for better patient experiences and outcomes.

The key, however, lies in getting clear about how far you're willing to go. This is your life, and you're the one who needs to live with your choices. No one else. So, you also need to get clear on why having a baby and becoming a parent is something you want. Above all, answer this important question: 'What is most important to me – the means of getting to baby or the baby?' This will help you get clarity on the choices available to you. Most of my patients report that, no matter what, doing what it took to become the best version of themselves through the application of the F.E.R.T.I.L.E. Method® (even when in some cases combined with other treatment options as well) was a key step on their journey – because they'll never have to live with the regret of wishing they'd done more. Applying a comprehensive strategy brought a sense of completion to their journey, regardless of the outcome.

• TAKE A BREATH •

And remember, any choice backed by even the beginning sketches of something resembling a plan is infinitely better than continuing to go around in circles until you run out of time altogether and are left wondering 'What could have been if I'd taken charge and made a choice?' If you fail to make a decision, life will eventually make it for you. Then, all you can do is adjust to what is.

References

1   Fontana, R., et al., The deep correlation between energy metabolism and reproduction: A view on the effects of nutrition for women fertility. *Nutrients*, 2016. 8(2).

2   Piché, M.-L.P., et al., Lifestyle-related factors associated with reproductive health in couples seeking fertility treatments: Results of a pilot study. *International Journal of Fertility & Sterility*, 2018. 12(1).

3   Salas-Huetos, A., et al., The effect of nutrients and dietary supplements on sperm quality parameters: A systematic review and meta-analysis of randomized clinical trials. *Advances in Nutrition* (Bethesda, Md.), 2018. 9(6).

4   Samkange-Zeeb, F.N., et al., Awareness and knowledge of sexually transmitted diseases (STDs) among school-going adolescents in Europe: A systematic review of published literature. *BMC Public Health*, 2011. 11.

5   Nyasulu, P., et al., Knowledge and risk perception of sexually transmitted infections and relevant health care services among high school students in the Platfontein San community, Northern Cape Province, South Africa. *Adolesc Health Med Ther*, 2018. 9.

6   Peterman, T.A., et al., Cumulative risk of chlamydial infection among young women in Florida, 2000–2011. *Journal of Adolescent Health*, 2014. 55(2).

7   Cha, S., et al., High rates of repeat chlamydial infections among young women – Louisiana, 2000–2015. *Sex Transm Dis*, 2019. 46(1).

8   Lee, D.-H., Evidence of the possible harm of endocrine-disrupting chemicals in humans: Ongoing debates and key issues. *Endocrinology and Metabolism*, 2018. 33(1).

9   Marques-Pinto, A., et al., Human infertility: Are endocrine disruptors to blame? *Endocrine Connections*, 2013. 2(3).

10   Wilcox, A.J., et al., The timing of the 'fertile window' in the menstrual cycle: Day specific estimates from a prospective study. *BMJ: British Medical Journal*, 2000. 321(7271).

11   Wilcox, A.J., et al., Post-ovulatory ageing of the human oocyte and embryo failure. *Human Reproduction* (Oxford, England), 1998. 13(2).

12   Kasius, A., et al., Endometrial thickness and pregnancy rates after IVF: A systematic review and meta-analysis. *Human Reproduction Update*, 2014. 20(4).

13   Dodge, L.E., et al., Women's alcohol consumption and cumulative incidence of live birth following in vitro fertilization. *Journal of Assisted Reproduction and Genetics*, 2017. 34(7).

14   Domar, A.D., et al., Lifestyle habits of 12,800 IVF patients: Prevalence of negative lifestyle behaviors, and impact of region and insurance coverage. *Human Fertility* (Cambridge, England), 2015. 18(4).

15   Firns, S., et al., The effect of cigarette smoking, alcohol consumption and fruit and vegetable consumption on IVF outcomes: A review and presentation of original data. *Reproductive Biology and Endocrinology: RB&E*, 2015. 13.

16   Grainger, D.A., et al., Preconception care and treatment with assisted reproductive technologies. *Maternal and Child Health Journal*, 2006. 10(Suppl 5).

17   Johnson, K., et al., Recommendations to improve preconception health and health care – United States. A report of the CDC/ATSDR Preconception Care Work Group and the Select Panel on Preconception Care. *MMWR. Recommendations and Reports*, 2006. 55(RR-6).

18   Kamphuis, E.I., et al., Are we overusing IVF? *BMJ (Clinical research ed.)*, 2014. 348.

19   Teoh, P.J., et al., Low-cost in vitro fertilization: Current insights. *International Journal of Women's Health*, 2014. 6.

20   Pilcher, G., 'Cost of raising a child to 18 is now $1 million, according to research.' 2009. Retrieved from https://news.com.au.

21   Capuano, G., 'Are children staying at home for longer?' 2017. Retrieved from https://blog.id.com.au.

22   Fry, R., 'It's becoming more common for young adults to live at home - and for longer stretches.' 2017. Retrieved from www.pewresearch.org.

23   Biggers, J.D. IVF and embryo transfer: Historical origin and development. *Reproductive Biomedicine Online*, 2012. 25(2).

24   Wang, J. et al. In vitro fertilization (IVF): A review of 3 decades of clinical innovation and technological advancement. *Therapeutics and Clinical Risk Management*, 2006. 2(4).

25   We are working with Harvard University and The University of Sydney Biostatistics Faculty to complete the retrospective analysis of The Natural Fertility Breakthrough Program™ patient data. Our patients are mostly over 40 and have been trying unsuccessfully to conceive or take a healthy pregnancy to term for over two years. For the patients who complete The Natural Fertility Breakthrough Program™, our overall success rate is 78.15%. This is an extraordinary result given that couples who undergo IVF/ICSI treatment typically see a 25–30% success rate. The full analysis and our official report will be published in early 2020.

Conclusion – From Beginning To Baby And Beyond

'Whatever your goal is you will never succeed
unless you let go of your fears and fly.'

Richard Branson

The truth is, you already know what to do.

You haven't had it easy, but one thing is for sure: the story you choose to write from this point is entirely up to you. Having read this book, you can no longer blame yourself, your partner or the circumstances. You now realise there are things you can influence and things you must accept.

So, knowing what you know now, will you choose to get serious and do what it takes, for as long as it takes, up to the line you drew for yourself, or not?

Here's another question: what story would you rather have read back to you when all is said and done – the story where you did whatever it took or the story where you gave up? This question guides my daily and seemingly insignificant habits, which, over time, come to represent major life choices.

The story where I make a choice, where I take charge, persist and conquer – that's a valuable story to me. That's the story I want read back to me. It's the story that continues to ignite my passion and drive on this journey called life.

Let it be the same with your story. You are your own hero. Don't underestimate this truth.

There is immense freedom in choosing to get off one train so you can catch another – one that's heading to your ultimate destination, no matter where that is.

If you decide you've given enough and no longer want to continue pursuing the baby dream, it's time to catch a different train. This means deciding to free yourself and your energy, so you can devote yourself to another cause or a different version of parenthood. This choice, like every other, requires courage, and making it means you're a true winner in your life. You're not a victim of your circumstances. You are an inspiration to yourself and others. You have decided to begin a new chapter. Good for you.

'You are braver than you believe, stronger than you seem, smarter than you think and loved more than you know.'

Christopher Robin, *Winnie the Pooh*

On the other hand, if you (like most of my patients) just know, in your heart and in your gut, that you're not yet done, then it's time for a new, holistic and more comprehensive strategy. It's time to stop doing the same thing while expecting a different result. It's time for deep and significant change that begins from the inside.

Decide which story you'd rather have read back to you and begin writing it now.

I believe wholeheartedly in your body's ability to adapt and regenerate when the obstacles to optimum health and fertility are identified and effectively addressed. I also know the answer to your fertility is not 'out there'. It's not a magic cure to be given by any practitioner treating you. It's inside. It's tucked away within your body's inner wisdom. It's waiting to be coaxed and rediscovered.

My team and I can guide, we can educate, we can cajole, but there comes a point when only you individually can do the work. Only you can choose to develop your determination. Only you can find your strength and take charge of your journey. Only you can write your story. It's only when you do your part that the Heavens will come to your aid. And even though the ultimate outcome may not be up to you, the deep, action-focused desire to make things happen cannot come from anyone or anywhere else other than you.

You are not alone. I believe in you. I believe in your abilities, and I truly believe you are whole just as you are right now. You are your own miracle. Nothing will change this truth.

Even if our paths never cross again, I want you to know that you are loved more than you'll ever know, and I hope that if nothing else, I have awakened in you this very simple truth. I wish you the very best on your fertility journey. Nothing else comes close to the feeling of fulfilment I experience when I witness the transformations I have helped spark into life in some way (especially when those transformations are 'our' babies). So, please do keep me posted on your metamorphosis. In the meantime, remember to keep the faith, do what it takes and enjoy the ride.

'Yesterday I was clever, so I wanted to change the world.
Today I am wise, so I am changing myself.'

Rumi

Take charge. Only you can.

Big love,

xg

P.S. This book is my love letter to you. If in any way I've helped you create your happy new beginning (whatever that looks like), please do reach out and let me know how via Facebook messenger at Facebook.com/gabriela.rosa.

Get In Touch –
Let Me Help You

If you've been trying to conceive for over two years and/or have experienced (recurrent) miscarriage, or you have three or more obstacles (aka minor factors) to optimum health and fertility and you've tried many treatments that haven't worked, it's likely you're still missing critical pieces in your fertility puzzle.

If you've been trying for a long time, further delay could mean running out of time to experience parenthood altogether. So, if you're feeling stuck, and we're a good fit for working together, my team and I would like to help you.

The Natural Fertility Breakthrough Program™ has an overall 78.15% success rate and is ideal for couples who are ready to stop going around in circles on their fertility journey.

If this is you, please contact my team for a complimentary conversation with one of our clinical assistants. If they believe you're the type of patient(s) we do our best work for, our team can guide you through the necessary steps, and I may even have the pleasure of personally assessing your case and helping you recreate your path to parenthood.

We treat patients all over the world, though limited appointment spaces are available. You can book an initial complimentary session or secure an obligation-free phone conversation with one of my team at http://thefertile.me/NFBPInfoSession.

I look forward to connecting with you, and in the meantime, I wish you the very best on your journey towards realising your dream.

Glossary

Adrenal insufficiency Adrenal insufficiency occurs when the adrenal glands don't make enough of certain hormones, including cortisol (sometimes referred to as a 'stress hormone')

ALS Ammonium lauryl sulfate

AMH Anti-müllerian hormone

APGs Alkylpolyglucosides

ART Assisted reproductive technology/treatment/techniques

ASI Adrenal stress index

BBT Basal body temperature

BCP Birth control pill

BFN Big fat negative

BPA Bisphenol A

Breakthrough An act or instance of moving through or beyond an obstacle

CAM Complementary and alternative medicine incorporates modalities of effective treatment used in evidence-based holistic and integrative medicine

DNA Deoxyribonucleic acid

Donor egg The use of another woman's egg to enable a woman or couple to conceive through ART

Donor embryo The use of a donated embryo to enable a woman or couple to conceive through ART

E2 Oestradiol

EDCs Endocrine-disrupting chemicals

Egg quality The state of a human egg being genetically normal or abnormal. Although this status is not always possible to specifically observe, signs that egg quality may be negatively affected may include inability to conceive, poor fertilisation rates or abnormal embryo development. Unlike ovarian reserve, egg quality can be improved (with the correct strategy)

Endometriosis A condition resulting from the appearance of endometrial tissue outside the uterus

Epigenetics	The study of heritable changes in gene function that do not involve changes in DNA sequence
Failed IVF cycle	Failure of an IVF/ART cycle to result in a successful pregnancy
Fertile Diagnostic Assessment™	A fertility assessment to specifically uncover impediments to optimum fertility conducted at the Rosa Institute
F.E.R.T.I.L.E. Method®	An effective seven-step process created by fertility specialist Gabriela Rosa to help couples overcome infertility and miscarriage, even when other treatments have failed. This method focuses on supporting couples (and individuals undergoing solo reproduction) from beginning to baby. The journey in steps includes: fact-find, educate, recommend, treat, incubate, liberate, and end result
Fertilisation	The fusion of male and female gametes to form a zygote
Fertility Challenge™	A proven online, interactive, educational and transformational two-week event created and hosted by fertility specialist Gabriela Rosa. This event has now educated and inspired over 100,000 people in 100+ countries towards their dream of becoming a parent
FET	Frozen embryo transfer
FSH	Follicle-stimulating hormone
Genetics	A branch of biology that deals with the heredity and variation of organisms
GMO	Genetically modified organism
GP	General practitioner
GSD	Get stuff done
hCG	Human chorionic gonadotropin
Heroin addict syndrome	Definition created by fertility specialist Gabriela Rosa to exemplify the effect of epigenetics on reproductive outcome and why some people can get pregnant despite engaging in health-damaging behaviour while a health focused individual may still struggle
Holistic medicine	Treatment of the whole person, taking into account body, mind, spirit and emotions, not only the symptoms of a disease
Homeostasis	A relatively stable state of equilibrium
Homeostatic Fertility Pendulum™	A metaphorical explanation of how biochemistry is epigenetically modulated

Hormonal imbalance	When there is too much or too little of one or more hormones in the bloodstream
ICSI	Intracytoplasmic sperm injection
Implantation failure	Failure of the embryo to implant onto the side of the uterus wall
Infertility	Inability to conceive after 12 months of unprotected sexual intercourse. May also encompass the inability to carry a pregnancy to term
Insulin resistance	Reduced insulin sensitivity by insulin-dependent cells
Integrative medicine	A therapeutic system which blends evidence-based CAM and conventional medicine
IUI	Intrauterine insemination
IVF	In vitro fertilisation
Klinefelter syndrome	A set of symptoms that result from two or more X chromosomes in males
Life Changer Method™	The three-step process coined by fertility specialist Gabriela Rosa to enable long-lasting habit change: face it, feel it, flow with it
Male factor infertility	Fifty percent of the cause of infertility in couples, where a male is unable to effect a healthy pregnancy
MEA	Monoethanolamine
Menopause	The permanent cessation of menstruation
Mindfulness	A mental state achieved by focusing one's awareness on the present moment
Minor factors	The seemingly minor obstacles that prevent successful reproductive outcomes
Miscarriage	Pregnancy loss that occurs before 20 weeks gestation
MTHFR	Methylenetetrahydrofolate reductase
Naturopathic medicine	A CAM modality that emphasises holistic medicine as the foundational treatment of disease
NFBP	Natural Fertility Breakthrough Program™, an evidence-based integrative medicine treatment for couples who wish to overcome infertility and miscarriage
NKCs	Natural killer cells
Oocyte	A cell in an ovary which may undergo meiotic division to form an ovum

Ovarian reserve	A wildly misused term to describe total ovarian reserve (total oocytes remaining) while in fact only measuring a pool of recruited oocytes in a current cycle with the aim to ascertain (likely incorrectly) a woman's remaining reproductive potential[1]
Ovulation	The discharge of a mature ovum from the ovary
Ovum	A mature female reproductive cell
PCOS	Polycystic ovarian syndrome
Perimenopause	The period of time 'around menopause', in which the body makes the transition to the end of a woman's reproductive years: menopause
PGD	Pre-implantation genetic diagnosis (term often used interchangably with pre-implantation genetic screening)
PGS	Pre-implantation genetic screening
Preconception health care	The period of holistic preparation for pregnancy including both prospective parents, with the intention to optimise the health of the future mother, father and baby
Quats	Quaternary ammonium compounds
RAIN	Four-step mindfulness process to expand self-awareness. It includes recognise, accept, inquire, and note or non-identify
RBC	Red blood cell
Recurrent implantation failure	Failure to achieve a clinical pregnancy after IVF transfer of at least four good-quality embryos in a minimum of three fresh or frozen cycles in a woman under the age of 40 years
Recurrent miscarriage	Three or more consecutive pregnancy losses
Reproductive toxicants	Chemical hazards that interfere with normal reproductive function
Rosa Fertility Diet	Fertility specialist Gabriela Rosa's dietary recommendations for couples undergoing treatment at the Rosa Institute
Semen	The male reproductive fluid that contains sperm
Semen analysis	Measures the quantity and quality of fluid (and contents) released during ejaculation
SLES	Sodium laureth sulfate

Sperm	The male reproductive cell: spermatozoa
Sperm count	Number of spermatozoa per ejaculate or measured amount of semen
Sperm DNA fragmentation	Abnormal genetic material within spermatozoa
Sperm morphology	Size and shape of spermatozoa
Sperm motility	Forward progression of spermatozoa
Sperm quality	An overall extrapolation of a man's reproductive cells' ability to effect a healthy pregnancy; taking into consideration various sperm health markers such as count, morphology, motility, fragmentation, vitality antibodies and more
Sperm vitality	Percentage of live, membrane-intact spermatozoa in semen
Steadfast	Firm in belief, determination or adherence
Stillbirth	A pregnancy loss that occurs at or after 20 weeks gestation
STIs	Sexually transmitted infections
Subclinical disease	An ailment that remains clinically undetected
TgAb	Thyroglobulin antibody
TPOAb	Thyroid peroxidase antibody
TRAb	Thyroid stimulating hormone receptor antibody
TRH	Thyrotropin-releasing hormone
TSH	Thyroid stimulating hormone
Unexplained infertility	The diagnosis given after excluding anomalies in semen analysis, ovulation, and tubal patency test through standard fertility evaluation. Standard assessments fail to identify clinical and subclinical abnormalities for up to 30% of couples (and possibly more), who then receive this diagnosis
WHO	World Health Organization
Y chromosome microdeletion	A host of genetic disorders caused by missing gene(s) in the Y chromosome

11 Pillars of Fertility Foundations™   The underlying premise upon which the F.E.R.T.I.L.E. Method® is based. The eleven areas include the Rosa Fertility Diet; personalised nutritional supplementation prescription; home and personal environment assessment and optimisation; fertility-boosting movement and exercise; male fertility and holistic reproductive health assessment and treatment; female fertility and holistic reproductive health assessment and treatment; decompressing and regulating stress for a fertile outcome; revitalising sleep, rest and relaxation strategies for optimum fertility; balancing whole body biochemical wisdom; accounting for mind over matter fertility mindset; and building family foundations from beginning to baby and beyond

References

1   Gleicher, N., et al., Defining ovarian reserve to better understand ovarian aging. *Reproductive Biology & Endocrinology: RB&E*, 2011. 9(1).

Acknowledgements

Mission accomplished – for now. And it's never the work of one person. The reality is that every single person with whom I have ever crossed paths in some way shaped the person able to put these words on paper. For each encounter, I am grateful.

To my many mentors over the years, thank you for helping me shine the light on that path less travelled, and for ushering the way. You have my unending love and gratitude.

Then there is my whole team at the Rosa Institute and the beautiful and 'ever ready to serve' moderators of my online programs (Susan, Ali, Stephanie, Natalia, Kristine, Karla). Without them, none of it would be possible. All of you guys are my heroes without capes (although, if you really want, I'll get some made up for you because you deserve it!).

Georgia, Susan, Alison and Ivy, without your unrelenting and uncompromising efforts in getting the manuscript together and/ or 'holding the fort' so I could disappear for days on end to finish writing this book, we would still be sitting on a first draft rather than the real thing. And to the entire Rosa Institute team – the amazing practitioners and administrative teams who take amazing care of our patients, and without whom none of it would be possible: you guys make dreams come true. A huge thank you for all of your efforts and also for being my partners in that little hallucination I have from time to time – the one where we make the world a better place, one healthier baby and family at a time.

To the team at Rethink Press – you guys took my little seedling of an idea, cultivated it, tended it and delivered this baby with the utmost professionalism and care.

Debbie, thank you for originally piecing my ideas together, especially when I felt it was all too hard. I am so grateful and look forward to many more books together.

To my family – you are the best, most unwavering cheerleading squad anyone could ever wish for. Your contribution to my life's mission will likely be unmatched in this lifetime. Mum and Dad, you guys are the absolute best example of disciplined, determined effort I could ever wish for. If ever I'm unsure about the enormity of any task, I just need to remind myself whose daughter I am and where I come from. If I am – half – as good a parent to my children, they will indeed be incredibly fortunate. Thank you.

Dani, thank you for the life lessons. I love you. Jayb you are still my fave. Maurice and my darling boys, Jake and Josh, *you* are my dreams come true.

And right up there with you are the strong and brave souls I'm truly honoured to guide on their journey to parenthood and making their own dreams come true – my patients. You guys continue to give me the greatest opportunity and one of the most precious gifts of my life – the chance to constantly evolve and to serve at ever-growing levels. Thank you. Always.

The Author

Gabriela Rosa MScM (RHHG), BHSc (ND)

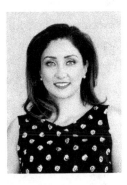

Gabriela Rosa is a world-renowned fertility specialist, host of The Fertility Challenge™ and the founder and clinical director of the Rosa Institute – an organisation dedicated to helping couples create healthy babies despite previous reproductive challenges.

Since 2001, Gabriela and her team of clinicians have been blending evidence-based science into a holistic, supportive and education-focused approach to fertility treatment, underpinned by her unique F.E.R.T.I.L.E. Method®. This proven and effective methodology is the underlying foundation of Gabriela's signature programs, which have now provided reproductive education and empowerment to over 100,000 couples in more than 100 countries worldwide.

Gabriela is the author of four books on natural fertility solutions, including two bestsellers. Her newest book includes essential information for couples who have struggled for over two years to conceive and/ or have had difficulty taking a healthy pregnancy to term. Gabriela has been featured in major media publications, including the *Daily Telegraph*, *Woman's Day* and *New Idea*. She is an inspiring and motivating educator as well as a popular podcast and radio commentator on the topics of natural health and fertility.

With the aim of advancing scientific knowledge through clinical fertility research, Gabriela has completed clinical research programs at Harvard University's T.H. Chan School of Public Health and was awarded the Scholar Award for academic excellence. Currently working towards a master's in public health, Gabriela already holds a Master of Science in Medicine (Reproductive Health and Human Genetics) from the

University of Sydney, a Bachelor of Health Science from The University of New England and is trained in numerous health disciplines, including naturopathy, nutrition and botanical herbal medicine.

Together with her team, Gabriela works diligently to provide couples with a science-based, holistic and integrative medicine approach to creating healthy families, despite the odds, one healthy baby at a time.

For updates on Gabriela's latest initiatives,
visit www.gabrielarosa.com

CPSIA information can be obtained
at www.ICGtesting.com
Printed in the USA
LVHW010800260620
658994LV00014B/2018